Healing Plants of Greek Myth

The origins of Western medicine and its plant remedies derive from Greek myth

Healing Plants of Greek Myth

The origins of Western medicine and
its plant remedies derive from
Greek myth

Angela Paine

MOON
BOOKS

Winchester, UK
Washington, USA

JOHN HUNT PUBLISHING

First published by Moon Books, 2022
Moon Books is an imprint of John Hunt Publishing Ltd., No. 3 East Street, Alresford
Hampshire SO24 9EE, UK
office@jhpbooks.net
www.johnhuntpublishing.com
www.moon-books.net

For distributor details and how to order please visit the 'Ordering' section on our website.

Design: Stuart Davies

UK: Printed and bound by CPI Group (UK) Ltd, Croydon, CR0 4YY
Printed in North America by CPI GPS partners

We operate a distinctive and ethical publishing philosophy in all areas of our business, from our global network of authors to production and worldwide distribution.

Contents

Other Books by Angela Paine

The Healing Power of Celtic Plants
Their history, their use, the scientific evidence that they work
ISBN 978 1 90504 762 8

Healing Plants of the Celtic Druids
Ancient Celts in Britain and their Druid healers
used plant medicine to treat the mind, body and soul
ISBN 978 1 78535 554 7

Acknowledgements

Firstly, I owe a huge debt to Rosie Wingate for her patient editing skills and John Daniell for his invaluable help with the botanical drawings. I'm grateful to Nimue Brown and the lovely Trevor Greenfield for their help and advice, always provided so quickly and with good humour. Thanks go to Petros Stergiou, who not only provided me with board and lodging while I was in Greece carrying out some of the research for the book, but also illuminated me on all things Greek during delightful evenings sipping Greek wine.

Abbreviations

m - metre
cm - centimetre
ml - millilitre
kg - kilogram
ppm - parts per million
PMS - pre menstrual syndrome
LDL - low density lipoprotein
HDL - high density lipoprotein

Part 1

Introduction

The original goddess religion of ancient Greece

In ancient times the area in the southern Mediterranean which we now recognise as Greece was a paradise of beautiful forested islands, rivers running down from mountain peaks, where animals large and small roamed and seas teamed with fish. No wonder this was one of the first places in Europe where humans chose to live, attracted by the rich vegetation and wonderful climate, feasting on the abundant fruit, meat and fish. They cleared little plots of land for crops and pasture, built houses and boats and used the plants around them as food and medicine. The ancient tribal hunter gatherers lived in small settlements, making little impact on their environment and worshipping many goddesses. The archeo-mythologist, Marija Gimbutas, spent years tracing the goddess culture of ancient, Neolithic Europe, including Greece, through photos and drawings of statues, carvings and decorative motifs on a multitude of different objects. Through these she was able to trace a matrilineal order of inheritance in the area. Inextricably intertwined with this goddess worship was a profound reverence for every aspect of the natural environment: the trees, flowers, herbs, animals, birds and fishes, as well as the rivers, streams and pools, the mountains and the sea. Many of the symbols Gimbutas discovered were abstract, representing a complex system of interlocking elements and people, suggesting that the ancients were aware of the interconnectedness of all life. She found goddess figures in tombs, temples, frescoes, reliefs, sculptures, figurines and paintings. The earth goddess was the universal fruitful source of all things and goddess religion lasted for a very long time, much longer than the male-dominated religions that came after, with the invasion of the Helenes.

Ancient goddesses were represented as naked, demonstrating

the powerful and dangerous sexuality of the divine female. The Mistress of the Animals, a naked goddess, was a common theme throughout the Eastern Mediterranean region and Mesopotamia, and she was later imported to Greece. Nanno Marinatos, in "the goddess and the warrior," suggests that the Mistress of the Animals transformed into many Greek characters: Medusa, the adversary and patroness of men; Artemis, patron of elite warriors in early Greek religion and Circe. Medusa was the initiator of young men, subjecting them to a violent initiation under the tutelage of Artemis, alter ego of the Gorgon/Mistress of the Animals. Circe, who features a combination of sexual appeal and danger, means 'she-hawk' in Greek and like the Mistress of the Animals, she was a hunter and both predatory and protective. She transformed her visitors into wolves and lions and kept them living tamely around her palace. In 600 BCE the Mistress of the Animals appeared in Crete as Potnia Theron, an Artemis-like goddess. This motif, which appeared in the Bronze Age, may indicate an earlier version of Artemis in the Mycenean era. It reappears in the 7th century BCE in central Greece, winged, un-winged and semi-winged.

Hera, wife of Zeus, demonstrated her powerful independence when she became pregnant from the milky white fluid in lettuce, which resembled semen.

In Plato's Banquet Aristophanes, talking about gender, says humans were originally divided into male, female and androgyne, a being who had male and female sex organs. They also had two bodies and two converse faces on the same head, were physically perfect and completely independent since they could reproduce alone. This image is reflected in the mediaeval alchemical androgyne, symbol of immortality, transcendence and triumph over deceptive duality, the ultimate goal of alchemy. In early Greek myth there are several instances of people changing sex: Maestra changed from a woman to a man, Tiresias and Sithon changed from men to women, Iphis changed from a woman into a man and Kainis, a man, changed into a woman. The god Hermaphroditos, son of Hermes the messenger and Aphrodite, had both sets of genitalia. He came by these in a curious manner. Born originally as a boy, when he grew up, he went to the woods near Halicarnassus where he met a nymph, Salmacis who lusted after him. He ignored her, took his clothes off and dived into a pool. She flung her clothes onto the ground, jumped into the pool and clung to him, shouting to the gods, begging them to join them together forever, which the gods did, thus transforming him into a hermaphrodite. He asked his parents to curse the pool so that anyone who bathed there would become like him.

The original myths and stories of these ancient Neolithic peoples were absorbed into the profoundly paternalistic myths of the invaders, changed and overlaid with conquering gods who chased and raped the mortal women and goddesses they desired. Zeus, a multiple rapist, did away with the androgynes by cutting them into their separate male and female parts. The first goddess to represent Mother Earth came to be known as Gaia, a female goddess who reproduced asexually. Centuries later Hesiod's Theogony related the story of her fertilisation by Uranus, her first born son, who raped her repeatedly. She gave birth to many children, including six Titans, six Titanids, three Cyclops and the three Hecatonchires, huge creatures with a hundred hands each. Uranus, afraid of his children, imprisoned them in Tartara, a cold, dark place in the depths of the earth. Gaia, who had never enjoyed being raped, finally decided to do something about it. She gave Cronus, her youngest son, a scythe with which to mutilate his father. That night Cronus cut off his father's genitals using Gaia's scythe. Gaia advised Zeus to release the Cyclops and Hecatonchires, who defeated the Titans and threw them into the earth.

According to Mariolakos Elias, professor of Geology at the University of Athens:

"The end of the Titans means:
i) a relative abatement of earthquakes and volcanic activity, and
ii) the end of the direct and decisive influence of the natural
environment in the life of prehistoric humans. It is the period when
the food-gatherers and hunters are turned into farmers and animal
breeders."

Supreme goddess Mother Earth was also called Hypertatan Gan by the early Greeks, who worshipped her as earth-chthon, a part of nature with its soil and underground, which feeds and sustains humans. Sophocles accused humans of hurting the goddess by:

"...ploughing (her body) with his plough, incessantly furrowing
her year after year."

Demeter, another pre-Hellenic goddess, was, according to Anna Maria Corradini, like Gaia, a parthenogenetic goddess, who produced the natural world and her daughter, Persephone spontaneously out of her own body. According to Rigolioso the myth of Demeter and Persephone was originally a female only mystery which derived from the Sumerian myth of Inanna, who chose voluntarily to descend into the underworld. The invading Helenes added layers when their male gods intruded violently into the story.

Inextricably interlinked with the disrespect for the goddess culture was a total disrespect for the natural environment. The invaders cut down whole forests of trees for carving, building, burning, making charcoal, mine props, and for building enormous war ships, fortifications, bridges and houses. By the time of Pliny (23 - 79 CE), who described trees and forests as the most important of all Nature's gifts to man, much of the beautiful landscape that the ancient Neolithic peoples enjoyed had been changed out of all recognition. Pliny lamented the loss:

"The forests were temples to deeds of valour. Statues of the gods in gold and ivory were not greater objects of veneration than trees."

Plato (428– 347 BCE ca) wrote despairingly of the lost beauty of Attica:

"What now remains compared with what then existed is like the skeleton of a sick man, all the fat and soft earth having wasted away, and only the bare framework of the land being left; there are some mountains which now have nothing but food for bees, but they had trees no very long time ago, and the rafters from those felled there to roof the largest buildings are still sound."

But many parts of the ancient world were still covered in dense forests. Theophrastus (371 – ca 287 BCE) spoke of the cypress, oaks, maples and plane trees that covered Crete, and Homer, the semi-legendary author of the Iliad and the Odyssey, describes Crete as a beautiful wooded island.

The Origins of Greek Medicine

Greek myth has not only survived up to the present day but is intertwined with the origins of Mediterranean medicine and the Mediterranean plants used to heal the sick. Greek myth has spread into many aspects of modern life; for example, the Latin names (binomials) of many plants derive from the Greek, such as *Achillea* after Achilles, *Artemisia*, *Iris* and so on, while concepts enshrined in the Hypocratic oath still influence medical doctors today.

The origins of Greek Medicine are lost in the mists of time, before the era of the written word. There was a great deal of trade in ancient times and both goods and ideas changed hands, including healing plant products, such as opium, myrrh and frankincense. Many of the original healers were probably women, who collected the plants, especially the roots, which they needed to heal the sick, in secrecy. Root cutters, as they were called, may have existed as long ago as Greek medicine, collecting herbs, flowers, leaves and bark, as well as roots. But with the invasion of the Helenes these women healers were demonised, transformed into witches and sorcerers.

In the few surviving lines of his lost tragedy, "*Rhizotomoi*" (root cutters) in the 4th century BCE Sophocles described Medea, naked and chanting as she collected the silvery secretion oozing from a plant root into a bronze vessel. He may well have been describing one of the root cutters of Greece, who, though possibly not naked, probably surrounded their craft with secrecy. Root cutters, like wild plant collectors the world over today, would have jealously guarded the location of the healing and poisonous plants which they collected. Healers in the ancient world used incantations as part of their plant collecting rituals and when healing their patients. Chiron, Asclepius, Circe, Melampus, Machaon and Podaleirios all formed part of the magical, mythical circle of root cutters, according to Marija Gimbutas in 1989. These ancient healers knew that the roots were one of the most medicinally important plant parts. Roots fulfil several functions for the whole plant which partially explains why plant chemicals have a tendency to collect and concentrate there. They anchor the plant, absorb water and other nutrients, store energy in the form of starches and fibre; they produce hormones involved in tissue production. The roots of some plants funnel growth-inhibiting chemicals into the soil around them to reduce competition. They also contain compounds that help defend against predators by making the plant unpalatable or even poisonous. Many of the world's best-known healing herbs are used in root form.

The Greeks of pre-history told and retold stories of goddesses and gods who used plants to cure the sick, but it was not until the 8th century BCE that Minoan and Mycenaean scribes began to write the myths down. Homer's Iliad and Odyssey, the works of Hesiod and the plays of Aeschylus, Sophocles and Euripides are important sources of the myths in which goddesses and gods cured the sick with plant medicine, ritual, incantation and ceremony. The Greek word *botane* derives from *bosko*: to feed or nourish. Later it came to mean herb or plant and *botanikos* was the adjective meaning 'of herbs' while *botanicum* referred to a book about herbs. Homer refers to herbs, flowers and magical plants. Aristotle and Thales recorded the names of plants but most of their work is lost. Then Theophrastus (372-287 BCE) described the plant world of Greece in his Enquiry into Plants. He collected information from woodcutters, beekeepers and collectors of medicinal plants and classified them according to their sap, roots, leaves, buds, flowers and fruits. He observed the separation of the two sexes in certain plants.

In ancient Greek, the word *pharmakon* meant a single herb, *pharmaka*: herbs or drugs in the plural. *Pharmakeia* covered drugs, potions and charms, including herbs, magic, witchcraft and the concoction of poisons. Historian Georg Luck stated that *pharmakis*

"...*became one of the standard words for 'wise-woman/witch'.*"

Healing goddesses, such as Hekate in Hesiod's Theogony, had *polypharmakos*: "knowledge of many drugs or charms." Hekate, goddess of fertility and abundance, helped the Olympic gods to defeat the Titans. By the time of Homer, the patriarchal culture of the invading Helenes could not tolerate the idea of a powerful and free woman, so goddesses of herbs and healing had been transformed into something far more sinister: witches, and in the case of Hekate, a dark goddess of the Underworld. Circe, originally renowned for her encyclopaedic knowledge of herbs, both healing and poisonous, had become a monster who brewed herbs into dark, forbidding concoctions to transform her enemies into animals.

Originally healing goddesses were beautiful, powerful, all-seeing and all-knowing. As in many other parts of the world, original tribal healing women shamans, who possessed an encyclopaedic knowledge of medicinal plants, were re-labelled sorceresses or witches, as patriarchal society took over. Along with the destruction of the environment, went the downgrading of women healers, who were driven underground to avoid persecution. They formed secret societies which the male-dominated societies feared, transforming them into old, ugly, malign figures, living on the edges of society, in poverty. Although many feared them a few people sought them out for their healing knowledge or for more nefarious reasons, for they had knowledge of poisonous plants and could mix up a deadly brew if asked. Ironically the English word pharmacist derives from the Greek word *pharmikis*, (witch or wise woman.)

Apollonius Rhodius, Valerius Flaccus and many others speak of the witch Medea, another daughter of Hekate, who was renowned for her skill in the use of magical herbs. Jason would never have been able to steal the Golden Fleece without Medea's help. She not only created an ointment to protect him from her father's fire breathing bulls, but provided him with clever advice. Jason had been commanded by Medea's father to sow dragon's teeth in a field. From these teeth would grow an army of sword-wielding warriors. She told him to throw a stone into the middle of the warriors so that they would fight each other to death. She then used a herbal potion to euthanise the dragon who guarded the fleece, thus enabling Jason to steal it. Later she restored Jason's father and the Hyades to youth by boiling them in a cauldron with magical herbs. Medea left her basket of Kolkhian herbs (herbs from west Georgia) on Mount Pelion where they sprouted for the use of the Thessalian witches. It was many centuries later that her demonisation took place with the addition of the story of her killing her children, and ironically this is the part which has become the most famous.

The goddess Gaia makes a reappearance in Hesiod's story of Kronos, who devoured each of his children as soon as they were born, until his wife Rheia gave him a baby-shaped stone, wrapped in swaddling clothes, in place of his youngest son, Zeus. He swallowed the bundle without suspecting anything and Rheia hid her son Zeus on the island of Crete. When he grew up, he visited the goddess Gaia, now a healing goddess, who gave him a herbal emetic. He secretly fed this to Kronos who then vomited his brothers and sisters.

By the time of Homer, the knowledge of herbal remedies no longer belonged primarily to the goddess. There were by now a whole pantheon of gods and goddesses of medicine.

Artemis

Artemis, already mentioned in her role as patron of elite warriors in early Greek religion, was goddess of the hunt, wild animals, the wilderness, fertility, good health, girls, young women, childbirth and virginity. She, like her twin brother Apollo, had powers to heal and to kill, to cause plague and inflict all manner of diseases. At least two festivals were celebrated in honour of Artemis: Brauronia and the festival of Artemis Orthia.

Apollo

Apollo, one of the first gods of healing, was also capable of creating diseases and plague. The story of Apollo is yet another example of the usurpation of the power of the goddess by the invading male dominated cults. Pytho was the ancient name of present-day Delphi, a hidden valley at the foot of Mount Parnassus. Gaea, (another name for the earth goddess) gave birth to a female child who had an oracle in Pytho. Over the course of the centuries the female oracle that people came to consult was gradually transformed into Python, a fire-breathing male snake-like dragon with a barbed tail. Apollo, who needed an excuse to kill the female oracle/Python, said that the dragon was destroying villages around the oracle, laying waste to crops and poisoning springs. This was why, he said, that he had come to kill this monster, later boarding a boat disguised as a dolphin, in order to take command of the ship's crew. He forced them to bring him back to Pytho, where he changed the name to Delphi (derived from the word "dolphin,") and dedicated the oracle to himself.

We know very little about Apollo's healing techniques, mainly that he terrified everyone, including the other gods, and visited the plague on whole armies: during the Trojan war he brought the plague to the Greeks. Then he guided Paris while he shot Achilles's heel and killed him. According to the Encyclopaedia Britannia, from the time of Homer onward Apollo was strict and aloof, the god of divine distance, who threatened from afar. People could only communicate with him through oracles, prophets or his father, Zeus.

His forename Phoebus means "bright" or "pure,"and Apollo represented the solar principle which can destroy as well as give life to the environment. In his favour, Apollo took care of Chiron, the poor abandoned baby centaur, and taught him how to use healing herbs.

Chiron

Chiron the centaur was born as a result of the rape of the beautiful nymph Philyra by Kronos, who transformed himself into a stallion when Phylyra transformed herself into a mare in an attempt to flee. This resulted in the birth of Chiron, a centaur, half man and half horse. Philyra took one look at her new born baby and abandoned him in disgust. Since neither of his parents were interested in the baby, Apollo decided to take care of him and taught him all that he knew about healing herbs. As an adult Chiron lived in a cave on Magnesian Mount Pelion, where he studied the medicinal herbs which grew around him.

He taught many heroes, including the famous Asclepius who lived with him as a child.

Chiron became a powerful mentor to the sons of kings and many of the most famous Greek heroes, including Jason (of the Argonauts), Achilles and Hercules. Hercules, who had the bad habit of tipping his arrows with the blood of the monster Hydra, accidentally wounded his friend Chiron. Chiron could not find a cure for his wound, which caused him severe pain and never healed.

In Astrology Chiron symbolises the wounded healer who must face his own feelings of low self-worth and inadequacy and learn to rise above them. In the end Chiron freed himself from pain by renouncing his immortality in favour of Prometheus, and was placed among the stars.

Asclepius

Homer was the first person to mention Asclepius, the physician, in the Illiad. He speaks of him as contemporary with Hercules, Theseus and Jason. Richard Caton, in 1900, describes Asclepius's supposed birthplace a few miles from Epidaurus, an idyllic setting in the Hieron valley, surrounded by wooded hills. Nestling in the hillside on one side is a hamlet called Koroni, which still commemorates his mother. High up on another hill a temple to Maleatean Apollo looks down on the valley.

According to one myth Apollo, his father, had intercourse with the nymph Coronis, a princess of Thessaly, who became pregnant. Apollo ordered a white raven to guard her, while he went back to the land of the gods, where she was forbidden to enter. Coronis, pregnant and lonely, fell in love with Ischys, a mortal man, and made love with him. The watchful raven flew to Apollo to relate her unfaithful deed. Apollo burst into a rage and emitting a fiery blast, scorched the feathers of the unfortunate bird, turning him black from that day onwards. He then sent his sister, Artemis, to kill Coronis. She built a funeral pyre and flung Coronis onto it. Apollo watched, appalled as the mother of his unborn child was being consumed by the fire, then plunging a knife into Coronis, he was able to deliver his son, whisking him away from the flames, unharmed. He carried his newborn son to Chiron the centaur, in his cave on mount Pelion, and asked him to bring him up.

Chiron taught the young Asclepius everything he knew about the healing properties of the plants which grew on the mountain. He taught him surgery, aphrodisiacs and incantations and Asclepius grew up to become the best and most renowned physician in Greece, even able to cure snake bite, the most difficult ailment of all. He was so skilful with healing herbs that he was described, in Pindar's Pythian Ode, half a century later, as:

"To each for every various ill he made the remedy, and gave deliverance from pain, some with gentle songs of incantation; others he cured with soothing draughts of medicines, or wrapped their limbs around with doctored salves, and some he made whole with the surgeon's knife."

After his death he was always depicted carrying a snake-entwined staff, an image that has been adopted by physicians throughout the world. The ancients revered snakes who lived under the ground, since the earth was the source of divine wisdom. The sacred serpent tunnelled underground, discovering the secrets of the roots she encountered and had the power to use them for the benefit of the patients who visited Asclepius' healing sanctuaries. Roots were immensely important in ancient Greek medicine since they were produced by the all-nurturing Earth Goddess and therefore provided healing for both body and soul. The ancients were aware too that the snake is able to fascinate its prey before it strikes by a kind of hypnotism, a gift valued by shamans, healers and hunters. Serpents are often associated with shamanic spirit-guides. For example, when South American shamans take ayahuasca to induce trance, they often have visions of serpents which grant the shaman the gift to see the cause of sickness and how it can be healed. Egyptian reliefs show the Uranus serpent, which granted pharaohs divine wisdom and protection. In India I have seen a local shaman feeding the sacred cobra which guarded an ancient cave painting.

In some traditions Asclepius married Hygeia, goddess of cleanliness, while in others she was his daughter. Alternatively, he may have married Epione, goddess of soothing pain. All of Asclepius's many children grew up to become physicians and healers, known as the Asclepiads. His son, Machaon, helped Menelaos when he was wounded in the Trojan War. His son, Telesphorus, was the god of convalescence. His daughters were: Iaso, the goddess of recuperation from illness, Aceso the goddess of the healing process, Aegle the goddess of the glow of good health and Panacea the goddess of the universal remedy. The physicians and attendants who served the god were known as the *Therapeutae* of Asclepius.

The goddess Athena was so impressed by Asclepius's healing craft that she gave him some magical Medusa blood as a present, telling him that it would restore life to the dead. On several occasions he used it, to the horror of Hades, God of the underworld, who was infuriated every time one of "his" dead souls returned to the world of the living. The dead, he thundered, belonged to him. He petitioned Zeus to put a stop to this iniquitous behaviour, so Zeus raised a thunderbolt and struck Asclepius dead. Zeus, like many fiery personalities, repented of his rash and hasty action, since Asclepius had been such a wonderful doctor. So, he turned him into the constellation Ophiochus, where he has remained ever since, shining down on us from the sky. Greek myth and Astrology are intertwined, many of the gods and goddesses finding a place in the night

15

sky, where they continue to govern our fate.

The myth of Asclepius is connected with the origins of medical science and the healing arts. Whether he ever actually existed or not, people believed that the very thought of him could cure them, so they began to build temples, Asclepeion, to honour him. The temples were healing centres with sanctuaries to the God Asclepius and dormitories, where the sick were encouraged to sleep, surrounded by non-poisonous snakes.

Snakes, as already mentioned, were associated with divine wisdom, which comes from the heart of the earth. Their habit of shedding their skins represented regeneration, rejuvenation, immortality and eternal youth. Snakes represented, and still represent, among shamanic healers in remote parts of the world, wisdom, knowledge, healing, and are often associated with spirit-guides. So, the snakes represented an important healing message for the sick in the dormitories. As they lay dreaming, the God came to them and told them how to be cured. The patient then related their dream to the Asclepeion priest, who provided both treatment and explanation of the dream. The most famous Asclepeia were at Epidaurus and Kos. Over time Epidaurus became an important centre of healing and the site of athletic, dramatic and musical games in Asclepius' honour.

The Asclepeion at Epidaurus

I decided to visit the Asclepeion at Epidaurus, catching a bus from Athens to Palea Epidaurus: the port. Flanked by two gulfs, the Saronic and the Argolic; the Epidaurus region is beautiful, with steep hillsides thickly covered in trees, where travellers can walk on footpaths along the slopes of Mount Arachnaion. There are beaches, creeks, sailing boats, fortresses, ancient roads with bridges and guard posts, tombs, Byzantine churches and impressive monuments.

The following day I woke to the sound of wind rattling the shutters. Then I heard the pattering of rain. Black clouds loomed overhead menacingly.

I waited in the drizzle for the 8.20 bus, which never came, so I walked wetly out of the town and attempted to hitch hike. Someone picked me up and took me part of the way, dropping me on a straight road, somewhere near the turn off to the Asclepeion. The rain stopped. People pointed up the hill so I set off, only to find that the track ended in dense undergrowth. I returned to the road and tried another path tramping along pathways into the hillside until I ended up yet again in deep impenetrable undergrowth. Finally, I realised that the way was along the road. All the previous signs were a hoax to entrap the unwary biker or hiker.

Innocent little fluffy clouds speckled a brilliant blue sky. Softly sculpted hillsides clothed in green, little grey green olive trees and larger, brilliant green, fluffy branched pines, usher the way to the sacred site along a straight road. I came to a row of tall, slender, dark green cypress trees, leading to a large cafe, chairs and tables spread out under the trees. I walked on, up the hill.

I reached the theatre which, even on this wet, windy, autumnal day, was spectacular, cut into the hillside with a beautiful backdrop of olive and oak trees. According to Pausanias it was built in the 4th century BCE and designed by Polykleitos. The front seats of honour had marble backrests. With fifty-five rows of marble seats and twenty-four lines of stairs, the theatre seated 12,000 spectators with a theatre building in front for the actors to display scenery and two giant gateways on either side of the stage building to let the spectators in. The stage was elevated twelve feet and the proscenium was originally enriched by splendid sculpture.

I climbed up the steep steps, until I came to the highest seats, where I found the ground behind the top of the theatre carpeted with nut brown acorns. The slender branches of the oak trees bent down to touch the ground, birds tweeted and the wind sang in the trees. From the top of the theatre there is a magnificent view of the landscape beyond the theatre: in the foreground are Greek pines, behind which silvery green olive groves stretch into the distance, climbing the lower parts of the gently sloping hills which rise to the left and right protectively. This was the perfect position for a theatre. I imagined patients who had trudged along pathways and goat tracks to seek a cure for their psychological distress would feel a peace and contentment seep into them as they sat in the theatre and participated in ceremonies with music, theatre and sacred dance. In ancient times these were important for health and healing.

I left the theatre and went to visit the *Xenon*, or dormitory, originally an enormous building, now only visible as a stone outline in the midst of sweetly smelling pines, one pine tree actually growing inside one of the dormitory rooms. It was roughly divided into four sections, with further subdivisions. Remnants of the columns were scattered among the other stones. The building was originally two stories high with rooms that surrounded courtyards. This suggested that richer people paid more for better accommodation, while the poor would probably have slept on the floor of the central courtyards, wrapped in their own sleeping cloth, much as Indian pilgrims do today. They may well have walked long distances with nothing but a water pot, a stick and a shawl to wrap themselves against the sun or to sleep in.

I came to the remains of a magnificent temple to the Egyptian gods, then to the Hestiatorian complex, built in 300 BCE. This was a banqueting hall with huge, imposing columns at the entrance. A central courtyard was surrounded by 16 Doric columns on each side forming colonnades, behind which were rooms of various sizes. Priests in the central courtyard, offered part of the sacrificial animal to the God Asclepius then gave the rest to the worshippers. Archeologists found remnants of couches, fires and food in the courtyard, suggesting that the worshippers ate there. Some may have paid extra for one of the private rooms behind the colonnade.

I walked on and came to the site of the bath house. Towards the end of the fifth century BCE, they built a bath for the worshippers. By the end of the 4th century BCE, they built a new water transport system from the mountains to the sanctuary, with a water pipe which ended in front of Asclepius's temple. This supplied a bronze fountain-statue of Asclepius holding a cup, from which the water flowed, channeling into the bath building.

Theodotus built the enormous temple to Asclepius in 375 BCE. When I came to it, there was not much left, for it was destroyed by fire at the end of that century and thieves dug up the area under Asclepius's statue, a pit with stone walls, where people put their offerings and payments. The statue was a magnificent ivory and gold creation, a combination known as chryselephantine, decorated with brilliantly coloured enamel and seated on an elevated throne. Asclepius held his rod in his left hand and stretched out his right hand towards a snake. The temple to Asclepius was at the centre of the sanctuary, at the termination of the road from the town of Epidauros, which passed through a monumental gateway, or *propylaia*.

Eventually I found the place where the worship of Asclepius first began, in the 6th century BCE. In prehistoric times people worshipped a chthonic nature goddess in this area. Apollo, who seems to have had a habit of displacing goddesses, replaced the goddess, setting himself up as Apollo Maleatas. In the 6th century BCE people gathered in the mountain sanctuary of Apollo Maleatas to worship Asclepius. As time passed the crowds grew too large for the narrow mountain sanctuary so they moved to a sacred spring in the valley. They sacrificed animals to the god, roasting them over a fire beside the spring. Then they purified themselves by bathing in the spring water, and lay down on the ground beside it to sleep and dream of the God Asclepius. They believed that the sacred water purified and regenerated them, and their prophetic dreams helped to answer the questions they brought with them.

The presence of a sacred spring and a constant stream of pilgrims would have attracted the attention of the local priesthood, who would have arrived at the site and begun demanding payment, which went, eventually towards the building of the *Abaton*. The *Abaton* was a series of buildings round a central courtyard, built round the ancient altar, formed by the accumulated ash of sacrificial animals. The shallow porticoes round the courtyard probably provided shelter for people consuming the flesh of the sacrificial animals. In later times the ashes were held together and preserved within a wall, probably to conserve the venerable remnants of the older Asclepius worship. By the 4th century BCE, the number of worshippers had increased still further and the ritual banquets were transferred to the *Hestiatorian*. As more and more people made the pilgrimage to the sacred site, and the offerings continued to accumulate, bathhouses, dormitories, temples and gymnasiums were built with officiating priests, who laid down strict laws: no one could seek a cure without first making payment and if anyone failed to pay, they would be punished by the god.

Healing Inscriptions or *Iamata* at Epidaurus

I came across a stone stele, a flat standing stone with an inscription (*iama*) on it. The inscription described one of the cures of the Asclepeion of Epidaurus. A man with a wound on his toe was in a terrible state when the temple servants transferred him and sat him on a seat. When sleep came upon him a snake came out of the *Abaton*. When he woke, he realised he was healed. He said he'd dreamed of a handsome youth putting a drug on his toe. The snake, sacred animal of the god, healed the wound of the sleeping patient while the patient dreamed that the god healed him.

Another inscription, the inscription of Pamphaes says:

> *"Pamphaes of Epidaurus, having a cancerous sore inside his mouth. This man, sleeping here, saw a vision. It seemed to him the god opened his mouth with his hand, took out the sore, and cleansed his mouth and from this he became well."*

There are about seventy of these healing inscriptions on four stone steles at Epidaurus, divided into two kinds: those which describe the symptoms of the sick and their miracle cures: these deal with a voluminous diversity of issues, mostly related to health; and those that describe people's emotions and reactions to the events that take place. The inscriptions which deal with the symptoms of the sick describe the personal history of each patient, the specific disease they suffer from, the god's intervention and the miraculous cure. There is frequent mention that the patient must pay the god for healing before treatment can begin, and that the god will punish those who don't pay. Some patients made *ex voto* plaques or statues in gratitude for their cure, presumably after having already paid.

The inscriptions conveyed the idea to the person reading them that the god Asclepius would very likely visit them in a dream. Three out of the four stele were placed near to the *Abaton*, at the entrance to the Asclepeion, to make sure that the arriving patients who could read would see them. They may have been inscribed to put patients' minds at ease, or there is always the possibility that the *iamata* were used as propaganda tools, increasing the sanctuary's renown, eventually attracting people from all over Greece. When Pausanias visited in the second century CE there were still six steles, inscribed with miraculous cures, dating back to the 3rd and 4th centuries BCE. Now there are four.

Museum at Epidaurus

As I entered the museum, I saw an array of medical instruments: knives, tweezers, needle-like objects, and many other things that I could not identify. Here was evidence that surgeons operated on their patients in the Asclepeion. Simple surgical cures did take place, with the help of soporific herbs, such as opium, which was given to the sufferers before the act of *"enkoimesis,"* (dream induction), according to Helen Askitopoulou in 2002. The poppy flowers which ornament the marble ceiling of a sanctuary building provide evidence that doctors used opium to facilitate surgical interventions.

I spent hours wandering about in the magnificent Asclepeion, piecing together the story of how it came into being, starting with the sacred spring in the 6th century BCE. The Asclepion began as a place where people came for miracle cures for body, mind and soul. It developed into a blatant money-making enterprise. However, gradually a real medical profession began to evolve, with the use of bronze instruments as well as the herbal potions which had probably always been prescribed, for the use of healing herbs is older than written records. These early physicians took the pulse of their patients. They measured the size, frequency, strength, speed, fullness, order, quality and rhythm of the pulse and used it as a tool for prognosis, much as the Ayurvedic doctors of India today, who measure six different pulses in order to diagnose the patient. They questioned their patients about their diet, for the first option for treating disease was through diet, then exercise, bathing and sleep. They recommended that anyone who was fat would limit themselves to one meal a day, while normal weight people should eat two meals a day. Fatness was thought to lead to infertility, for the diversion of more food to make more body fat meant less food was available to produce menstrual blood which they thought was the raw material for a foetus. They also thought that a fat woman would be unable to support a foetus to full term. Galen's thinning diet included such foods as garlic, onions, cress, leeks and mustard because sharp, hot, biting foods could cut through the thick humours of the body.

Food has power: *dynamis* in Greek. This will become apparent throughout this book, where I list the healing properties of numerous foods which grew (and grow) in Greece. The ancient Greeks also made use of many healing herbs. Digestion was seen as a key process in the body, harnessing its natural heat to 'cook' the food into blood.

In ancient Greece health was seen as a balance of different fluids in the body as well as the way that the body related to the environment. Illness was thought to result from failure to honour the gods in the appropriate manner, so although the physician advised changes in diet, exercise and so on, the patient may also have had to pay a priest to make sacrifices or perform ceremonies.

Aristotle in his Nicomachean Ethics talked of the need for a golden mean or middle ground between deficiency and excess. And he was not just talking about food but morality as well. For this reason, athletes were not considered to be ideally healthy. "The athletic state," said Hippocrates in Nutriment, "is not a natural state; better the healthy condition."

Over 200 sacred therapeutic centres claimed that they'd been founded by the sanctuary of Epidaurus.

In the afternoon the sky clouded over, and the wind came rushing down the hillside with a burst of horizontal rain. The storm that swept in in the afternoon darkened the skies and raged through the Asclepeion transforming it into a dark, forbidding place, lashed by torrential rain and huge gusts of wind. The rain pelted down and ran in streams along the pathways.

Hippocrates

Hippocrates, who lived approximately between 460 - 375 BCE, during Greece's Classical period, appears to have traveled widely in Greece and Asia Minor, practicing his art and teaching his pupils. He was described by his younger contemporary Plato as "the *Asclepiad* of Kos," meaning a hereditary physician with a philosophical approach to medicine. Plato was the only near contemporary to write anything about Hippocrates, about whom very little is actually known. He was revered for his ethical standards in medical practice and supposedly said:

"In every house where I come I will enter only for the good of my patients, keeping myself far from all intentional ill-doing and all seduction and especially from the pleasures of love with women or with men, be they free or slaves."

His personality was constructed from the *Corpus Hippocraticum*, a collection of medical works put together by the Museum of Alexandria during the Hellenistic period about a century after his death. What survives of the *Corpus* consists of about sixty medical writings of different length and literary quality, written in different styles and expressing different points of view. Although attributed to Hippocrates, most were probably not written by him, but all are simple and direct, without technical jargon or elaborate argument. Some were clearly written in later periods. The works came to define ancient Greek medicine as practiced by Hippocrates and other physicians of his era and all agree on what disease is. Hippocrates' reputation, and myths about his life and his family, began to grow in the Hellenistic period.

According to Lloyd in 1978, Hippocratic medicine was based on the natural philosophy the Greeks had been developing since 500 BCE, at the time when vast numbers of people were visiting Asclepeia to seek miracle cures. Hippocratic doctors used careful observation, logical deduction, experimentation and record keeping. They were cautious and sceptical of the sacrifices and rituals carried out by the priests in the Asclepeia, preferring to observe their patients carefully, diagnose the cause of their illness and prescribe herbal cures or surgery. From the collection of surgical instruments that I saw in the museum at Epidaurus it is clear that Hippocratic doctors began practicing within the confines of the sanctuary at the same time as patients slept with snakes and dreamed of Asclepius.

The *Corpus Hippocraticum* describes symptoms, prognoses, and treatments for all parts of the body from the head to the feet. The medicine depends on a mythology of how the body works and how its inner organs are connected. There are works on diseases of women, childbirth, and paediatrics. Purgatives are prescribed to rid the body of the noxious substances thought to cause disease. There was no systematic research or dissection of human corpses at this time so, while much of the writing seems wise and correct, there are large areas where much is unknown.

The *Epidemics*, one treatise from the *Corpus*, lists annual records of weather and associated diseases, along with individual case histories and records of treatment, collected from cities in northern Greece. Diagnosis and prognosis are frequent subjects. Other treatises explain how to set fractures and treat wounds, feed and comfort patients, and take care of the body to avoid illness.

A number of the Hippocratic treatises deal with *Materia Medica*, composed of medicinal plants, but none of the Hippocratic writers attempted a systematic study of plant taxonomy.

Hippocratic physicians learned about aromatic baths from the Egyptians and developed teachings about using water as a form of treatment, which they called *hydropathy* or *thalassotherapy*.

Dioscorides recommended aromatic baths to treat urological and genital disorders, as well as for tumours, wounds, colds, bad mood, and fatigue.

According to Alakbarov in 2003 people have been using herbal baths since ancient times in the near east and the Mediterranean.

Bathing relieves muscle tension, dilates blood vessels and slows the heart rate. Many herbs give off their healing aromas when they are added to hot water thus reducing or eliminating mental and physical stress and benefiting hair and skin. Volatile oils are not the only agents working in an aromatic bath. Fragrant plants contain all sorts of other constituents, such as tannins, flavonoids, alkaloids and so on, that are also therapeutic. The infusion of the whole herb is often more effective than the pure volatile oil.

The Hippocratic oath

A committee founded the origins of medicine and medical ethics in Greece under the name of Hippocrates. Most of the original Hippocratic oath was a code of ethical principles concerning the ways in which physicians should teach each other's sons without charge and how the students should take care of their old teachers. The oath was edited to fit different societies as generations of physicians handed down fragments in various versions. The Hippocratic oath states that the physician pledges to prescribe only beneficial treatments, according to his abilities and judgment; to refrain from causing harm or hurt; and to live an exemplary personal and professional life. The Hippocratic oath was adopted as a guide to conduct by the medical profession throughout the ages and is still used in the graduation ceremonies of many medical schools.

Theophrastus

Theophrastus wrote his *Historia Plantarum*, between 350-287 BCE in ten volumes, of which nine survive. It was one of the most important books of natural history written in ancient times. He attempted a botanical classification based on plant structure, reproduction and growth. In book nine he covered the medicinal uses of plants, how to gather them, how to make juices, gums and resins, and how to use them to heal people. For example, he talks of the resin collected from the Aleppo pine, the pitch from the Corsican pine, gums such as frankincense, myrrh and balsam of Mecca, which are collected by making cuts in the trees. He appears to encourage euthanasia, saying that Hemlock will help bring about an easy and painless end. He advised people not to take any drug habitually since it would gradually cease to have any effect, advice that we should all take note of. Theophrastus had great respect for the powerful properties of plants and he understood that different healing plants may have many different properties and yet produce the same overall effect. He also understood that different people reacted differently to the same drug.

He described the practices of root cutters and plant collectors:

"Others say that cinnamon .... grows in deep glens, and that in these there are numerous snakes which have a deadly bite; against these they protect their hands and feet before they go down into the glens, and then, when they have brought up the cinnamon, they divide it in three parts and draw lots for it with the sun; and whatever portion falls to the sun they leave behind. And they say that as soon as they leave the space they see this take fire. Now this is sheer fable."

Stories about snakes were designed to discourage anyone who might decide to collect the herbs, barks, resins or roots for themselves.

He continually revised his manuscript, presumably as he discovered new information, so it remained in an unfinished state when he died. It was not until 1483 that a Latin translation by Theodorus Gaza was published. This was followed by Johannes Bodaeus's edition in 1644 to which woodcut illustrations were added. But English readers had to wait until 1916 for Sir Arthur Hort's English translation to be published.

Crateuas

Crateuas, who lived in the first century BCE, was another root cutter and personal physician, to Mithridates the 6th, King of Pontus, who lived in fear of being poisoned, since he was constantly at war with Rome. Crateuas created a poison antidote called *mithridatum*, a marvellous concoction of herbs and honey. According to Stephanie Pain in 2007, mithridatum was considered a cure for every illness for two millennia. It had such a reputation and was so expensive that apothecaries had to prepare it in elaborate public ceremonies in case they were tempted to leave out a vital ingredient.

According to Pliny, Crateuas produced a herbal with the earliest known coloured botanical illustrations. He classified the plants he described and explained their medicinal use. Unfortunately, his book did not survive but Dioscorides managed to copy some of it.

Dioscorides

Dioscorides, who lived from 40-90 CE, was a doctor who travelled extensively, studying the medicinal plants used by local people wherever he went and making careful notes. At least forty of the herbs he wrote about are listed in modern European pharmacopoeias. Many of the Greek plant names he mentioned have become modern botanical names. For example: Greek *anemone*: *Anemone species*; Greek *akoniton*: *Aconitum napellus*; Greek *smilax*: *Smilax aspera*; Greek *agnos*: *Vitex agnus castus*; Greek *krokos*: *Crocus sativus*; Greek *heliotropion*: *Heliotropium europaeum* and so on.

Dioscorides, probably incorporated much of Crateuas's herbal, together with some of Crateuas's illustrations, into his famous *De Materia Medica*. He compiled, organised, and published the most comprehensive pharmacological text in the ancient world with accounts of over 600 plants, their features, distribution and medicinal properties. *De Materia Medica* was copied many times, over the centuries. The most impressive copy was the richly illustrated *Codex Vindobonenesis* (512 CE), a Byzantine version of his herbal, made in Constantinople for a Byzantine princess. Herbalists and physicians used his work as a standard reference for hundreds of years.

Galen

Galen, who lived between 129 and 216 CE, was one of the most famous Greek physicians who influenced medical theory and practice in Europe until the mid-17th century. He studied medicine at Pergamum, Anatolia, part of ancient Greece and the site of a magnificent shrine to Asclepius. Galen spent much time dissecting animals, in order to improve his surgical skills and for research purposes. He was an accurate observer and distinguished seven pairs of cranial nerves, described the heart valves and observed the structural differences between the arteries and veins. Unfortunately, he did occasionally make mistakes due to the fact that Roman law prohibited the dissection of human cadavers at that time. But he influenced the development of anatomy, physiology, pathology, pharmacology and neurology in Western Europe. His written output was so enormous that his surviving writings represent nearly half the literature of ancient Greece. Many of his works are included in the Thesaurus Linguae Graecae, a digital library of Greek literature started in 1972. According to van Der Eijk in 1992, he brought together ideas from Hippocratic medicine and the philosophy of Plato and Aristotle to create an original synthesis that went on to dominate western medical theory and practice for many centuries. He took from Plato the idea of three organs, each in charge of an aspect of the body's functions. The brain controlled the nerves, arteries took one kind of blood from the heart to the rest of the body and veins carried nourishment from the liver to the rest of the body. He took from Aristotle the idea that nature does nothing in vain.

Galen was a workaholic, getting up at sunrise, attending the sick, frequently spending the night in study, even treating patients who lived-in far-off countries by correspondence. Many of his works were written in order to glorify his own skill. Interestingly he did not repudiate dreams as diagnostic instruments but rather interpreted them. His approach to his patients was thorough, taking notes on their age, temperament, complexion, temperature, posture, pulse, habits, activities, character, sex, and the region they lived in as well as the season and climate of that region. Location was considered important since climate and situation affect health and character.

Pliny the Elder

Pliny the Elder (23-79 CE) recorded the works of more than 400 authors and 2,000 manuscripts concerned with various aspects of the natural environment in his Natural History, thus saving them from oblivion.

Part 2

Sacred Trees
in Ancient Greece

When the Goddess culture prevailed, the lives of the people were inextricably intertwined with those of the trees and smaller plants that surrounded them. Originally people believed that trees were living, sentient beings, who communicated with those who could tune in to them. Then gradually as myths began to be recorded, tree spirits, in the form of Dryads and Hamadryads, began to separate from them. But the bond was still strong so that if either the Dryad was killed or the tree felled, the other half of the pair died. According to Athenaeus the forest-spirit Oxylos (of the forest) and the nymph Hamadryas (one with tree) lived on Mount Oita in Northern Greece. They may have presided over specific trees, for oxua in Greek can mean either woodland or beech tree and dros can mean holm oak or just tree. They were the parents of eight Dryad daughters, the Hamadryades: Kraneia, the nymph of the cornelian cherry tree, Aigeiros, the nymph of the black poplar, Ampelos, the nymph of the vine, Bryony, the nymph of black bryony and wrack (Fucus volubilis), Balanis the nymph of the holm oak and prickly-cupped oak, Karya, the nymph of the hazel nut tree, the walnut tree and possibly the chestnut, Morea the nymph of the mulberry tree, Ptelea the nymph of the elm tree and Syke the nymph of the fig tree.

By the late fifth century BCE the Goddess religions had been absorbed by God-based religions. I saw bas reliefs of Pan's nymphs in the Archeological Museum of Athens, looking demure in their voluminous robes, while Pan and the other gods sported fine naked torsos. This is a far cry from the magnificent Neolithic marble statues of naked goddesses who stood alone in the same museum, with no need of a male God. The Museum states that:

"...the nymphs were daughters of Zeus and goddesses of nature and they lived near springs in mountains through which rivers flowed, and in woods. Because of their close connection with water,

a fertilising element, they were worshipped as daemons of fertility and vegetation. They protected plants and animals and at the same time were Kourotrophoi (nurses), who occasionally also raised humans."

By the time myths were recorded there were numerous incidences of both human women and goddesses being transformed into trees to protect them from the ravishes of men, a poignant reminder that the Goddess religions were subjugated to the male-dominated religions of the warring invading tribes. Trees could weep, as the trees on the Canary Island of Tenerife still do today, letting fall a continuous shower of water drops, condensed from the encircling clouds, replenishing the underground water supply. But even after the Goddess religions had been subsumed into the patriarchal religion of Greek myth and the gods had been placed on Mount Olympus, in their palaces in the gorges – or 'folds of Olympus' as Homer calls them, there were still many species of sacred trees, most of which still grow on Mount Olympus.

Valonia Oak (*Quercus ithaburensis macrolepis*) Holm oak (*Quercus ilex*), Kermes oak (*Quercus coccifera*), Greek strawberry tree (*Arbutus adrachne*), prickly juniper (*Juniperus oxycedrus*) manna ash (*Fraxinus ornus*), smoke tree (*Cotinus coggyria*), Montpellier maple (*Acer monspessulanum*), Judas tree (*Cercis siliquastrum*), and turpentine tree (*Pistacia terebinthus*) grow on the lower parts of the mountain. Higher up there are montane conifers, such as black pine (*Pinus nigra var. pallasiana*), beech (*Fagus sylvatica*), Bosnian pine or black pine, Macedonian fir (*Abies borissi-regis*), oriental hornbeam (*Carpinus orientalis*), wych elm (*Ulmus glabra*), hazel (*Coryllus avellana*), dogwood (*Cornus mas*) and yew (*Taxus baccata*). In the gorges and ravines oriental plane trees (*Platanus orientalis*) and willows (*Salix eleagnos*) grow. From 1,400 to 2,500 metres altitude a rare species of pine, Bosnian pine (*Pinus heldreichii*) dominates. Some trees, such as the almond tree, are not native to Greece, but were adopted long ago and figure prominently in Greek myth. Many of the sacred trees of Greece have healing properties.

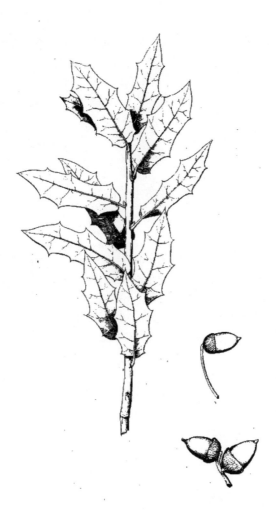

Oak Valonia *Quercus ithaburensis macrolepis*

Mythology

The Valonia oak at Dodona was the most ancient sacred tree in recorded Greek history. It was growing there in prehistoric times, during the era of goddess worship, when the earliest inhabitants of Greece, the Pelasgians, an ancient tribal people, were living there. The Valonia oak has big, edible acorns, which are low in tannin and the Pelasgians lived on them. Much later, in historic times people used to leach the tannin from the seeds by burying them in boggy ground over winter. The germinating seed was dug up in the spring when it would have lost most of its astringency. Whether the Pelasgians bothered to leach the tannin from the acorns before they ate them, we will never know.

The myth of the origin of humans begins with King Deucalion and his queen Pyrrha, who floated in a boat on the deluge for nine days, then came to rest on Mount Tomaros in Epirus, from which they threw stones which became men and women: the Pelasgians. Herodotus says:

"The Pelasgians were an ancient race widely spread over Greece, and the coast and islands of the Aegean Sea in prehistoric times: and traces of them are found in Asia Minor and Italy..."

Herodotus is pretty scathing about the Pelasgians, calling them barbarous and implying that when the Hellenes overran them, obliterating their language and many of their customs, this was a good thing.

According to Herodotus the prehistoric site at Dodona probably existed since about 2000 BCE. This was long before Zeus came to be associated with it, according to Peter Levi. Trees were particularly sacred because their roots went down into the ground and connected with the under-world, the mysterious abode of departed spirits, who were wise with knowledge of the future. The oak tree at Dodona had special prophetic powers because its roots pierced the earth more deeply than those of other trees, reaching all the way down to Tartarus. Strabo said in his Geography:

"A sacred oak tree is revered in Dodona, because it was thought to be the earliest plant created and the first to supply men with food."

In pre-Hellenic matrilineal Greece trees were alive with a supernatural essence. People who spoke the language of the spirit of the tree, who tuned in to the rustlings of the branches, could interpret the messages the tree wanted to convey. They interpreted the eerie sounds of the incessantly murmuring leaves stirred by the unceasing winds. Originally the tree was the spirit and only later did the all-knowing, prophetic doves, omens of death and spirits of the dead, who lived in the hollows of the ancient oak, become its indigenous spirits.

According to Pausanias:

"...the people in that part of the world... thought the most truthful oracles came from the wild doves and the oak trees..."

Herodotus of Halicarnassus asserted that Dodona was:

"...the most ancient and, at that period, the only oracle in Greece."

But who knows whether he was right, or whether, in fact, there were numerous other tree oracles which were simply not recorded?

When the Hellenes invaded, they transposed their god Zeus into Dodona, in a most uncomfortable position: "Not in the canopy of the oak tree...did the god dwell but on its floor," [*en pythmeni phegou*], according to Carl Kerenyi's translation of Hesiod. Zeus's prophets, the *Selloi*, slept on the ground under the sacred oak to listen to the roots of the tree and interpret what they had to say. The *Selloi* controlled the weather, enshrouding the tree in mist and settling down for the night in the fading light like ground-feeding doves. As the tree branches rustled, they disappeared into their earthy beds to experience prophetic dreams. It was a common practice in the ancient world, to sleep on sacred ground in order to incubate dreams and draw oracular wisdom from the earth.

The doves sat among the whispering leaves of the revered prophetic oak. They interpreted the rustling leaves as they sheltered from the wind in its hollow trunk and interpreted the meaning of the dreams of those who slept on the earth. Later, wise old women, ancient priestesses of Dodona, became what the Greeks called *oionomanteis* or, 'those who divined from birds.' The earliest works of Hesiod and Homer, as well as those of Sophocles, Aristophanes, and other later poets of the stage, are full of examples of people who divined from birds.

"For the ancient Greeks all birds were ominous and the word 'bird' itself was synonymous with omen as Aristophanes says."

Jane Ellen Harrison explains how people divined from birds, in her discussion of Hesiod's Works and Days. She comments that:

"...first and foremost you should watch the birds who are so near the heavenly signs, the teirea, and who must know more than man. This watching of the birds we are accustomed to call the 'science of augury'...in its origin it is pure magic, 'pure doing; the magical birds make the weather before they portend it."

The Greek phrase for observing "the heavenly signs" is *ornithas krinon*, which Harrison translates as "knowing in birds". The ancient people of Dodona sought advice directly from the doves and the tree and it was only later that the invading Hellenes established a formal oracle there.

After Zeus was appointed God of the sacred oak, priests collected money from those who came to seek answers to their questions and with this money they built a temple. There was an enormous gong outside the temple "which they say sounds all day if a passer-by lays a finger on it." Later this was replaced by a series of bronze cauldrons that formed a circle round the perimeter of the sacred ground. The endlessly echoing vibrations stirred by untiring winds, acted as a sound barrier that formed a magical circle of protection. Dodona became an important pilgrimage site.

The earth goddess appears to have held her own for many centuries after Zeus's usurpation. Pausanias speaks of a wise old priestess of the Dodona oak, called Phaennis, born in about 280 BCE and apparently "a member of a guild of sacred prophetesses called the Rock pigeons." He tells us that Phaennis, . . . and the Rock-pigeons at Dodona gave oracles from the god.

In 219 BCE, the Aetolians sacked the temple buildings at Dodona, then set about rebuilding them, but in 167 BCE the Romans destroyed them once again. The sacred oak survived and Pausanias said that it was still alive in the reign of Hadrian [117-38 CE]. Mrs Philpot informs us that:

"A later writer states that the oracular voices ceased on the felling of the tree by a certain Illyrian bandit... but there is evidence that the tree and the oracle were still in existence in the middle of the 4th century CE."

Over the centuries the most sacred tree in Greece bore witness to the building of temples and to their repeated destruction until eventually the Christians destroyed it. Prior to its murder, this ancient oak had stood, speaking its messages in the wind, for many more than 2,500 years. Howard Freemont Stratton wrote in 1937:

"Dodona has now lost its forest covering. The prophetic oak is gone. The miraculous spring that gushed from its roots has gone. The doves have gone. All trace of the sacred enclosure is gone. Hardly any trace of the temple remains."

The oak appears in many other Greek myths, such as the one about Biblis, a Miletian princess who fell in love with her brother. According to Antoninus Liberalis, and Ovid, when he rejected her advances, she fled in shame, and threw herself off a mountainside. The Nymphs pitied her fate and transformed her into a holm oak Dryad. Her tears became a spring which rose from the tree's roots. According to Athenaeus, Hamadryas Balanos was an acorn hamadryad.

According to Apollodorus, Apollonius Rhodius and Valerius Flaccus, the golden fleece was nailed to the branches of an oak tree in the sacred grove of Ares at Kolkhis. The god sent a giant serpent (*drakon*) to guard it.

According to Hunter in 2008, Erysichthon once ordered all trees in Demeter's sacred grove to be cut down. One huge oak was covered with votive wreaths, a symbol of every prayer Demeter had granted, so the men refused to cut it down. Erysichthon grabbed an axe and cut it down himself. As the dryad nymph was dying, she cursed Erysichthon. Demeter heard the nymph's curse and punished him by entreating Limos, spirit of insatiable hunger to put herself in his stomach. Erysichthon sold all his possessions to buy food but was still hungry. Eventually he sold his daughter Mestra into slavery. Poseidon freed her and gave her the gift of shape shifting into any creature. This enabled her father to sell her repeatedly, but he was still hungry. Eventually he ate himself.

Botanical Description

The oak was the dominant tree of the ancient Greek landscape. In fact, the ancient Greek word for oak, *'drys'*, was also the word for tree. *Quercus* species have alternate, simple, deciduous or evergreen leaves with lobed, toothed, or entire margins. The male flowers are borne in pendent yellow catkins, appearing with or after the leaves. Female flowers occur on the same tree, singly or in two to many-flowered spikes; each flower has a husk of overlapping scales that enlarges to hold the acorn, which matures in one to two seasons. The two main species of oak in the region are the evergreen holm oak and the deciduous Valonian. Both range in size from thick low shrub (forming the basis of the modern-day Mediterranean scrub forests) to large trees. The evergreen holm oak has shiny, dark green pointed leaves that are slightly toothed like holly.

The Valonian oak is a deciduous tree growing up to 15 m high and 13 m wide, often with a gnarled trunk and branches. The leaves are 4-9 cm long and 0.8-2.0 cm wide, oval with 7-10 pairs of teeth along a slightly carved margin. They are dark glossy green above, grey and hairy underneath. The male flowers are light green 5 cm long catkins while the female flowers are small, less than 0.4 cm, produced in 3's on short stalks and are wind pollinated. The acorns are generally oval, up to 5 cm long and 3 cm wide with a cap covering roughly 1/3 of the acorn, maturing in 18 months, dropping from the tree in the second autumn after pollination. The cap is covered in long stiff loose scales which are rolled backwards, especially along the edges of the cap. People extracted tannin from the acorn cups of the Valonian oak and used it to tan leather hides.

Healing Properties

Oak bark preparations are astringent, local anaesthetic, anti-inflammatory and bring down fevers. When applied to burns and wounds, oak bark infusions form a protective layer which allows the damaged tissues to heal and since they are anti-bacterial and anti-fungal, they will prevent wounds from becoming infected. They soothe gastritis and ulcers and cure mild diarrhoea. Gargling with an infusion of oak bark alleviates a sore throat.

Oak bark contains 8-20 % tannins. For a list of the chemical constituents of oak bark, and research that has been carried out on it see my book "Healing Plants of the Celtic Druids." No one has yet carried out any clinical trials on oak bark, but the European Medicines Agency came to the conclusion that it is safe, especially at therapeutic doses and concentrations, if only used over short periods.

How to Use

Take an infusion to treat diarrhoea, use as a mouth wash for minor inflammation or apply to the skin to soothe irritation. Use oak bark infusions to wash wounds and burns. Oak bark ointment is very effective for relieving the itching and burning of haemorrhoids. If you suffer from painful haemorrhoids you should always see a doctor before starting to use the oak bark ointment, just to make sure that you are not suffering from a serious condition.

Make a sitz bath with a quart of oak bark infusion to treat vaginitis: sore, inflamed vagina, which may be due to bacteria which cannot be detected, or too much sex. The oak bark will kill the bacteria, ease the pain and inflammation and tone the tissues. Use an oak bark sitz bath to ease haemorrhoids, fistulas and chronic pelvic pain.

Take half a cup of oak bark decoction three times a day to shrink goitre, reduce glandular inflammation, restore loss of voice and ease coughs, dry up mouth sores and bring down fever. Use oak bark decoction as a hair rinse to remove dandruff and encourage hair growth. Add oak bark decoction to your bath to heal varicose veins.

Contraindications

A few people are allergic to oak bark and oak pollen. Do not use oak bark during pregnancy and lactation. Provided it is not used over long periods and only in the recommended dosage, oak bark is safe. If taken together with other herbs it may interfere with the uptake of alkaloids and it might inhibit iron absorption.

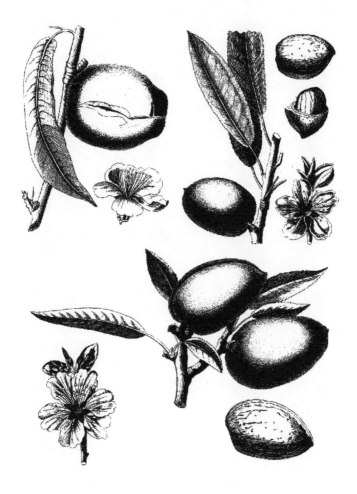

Almond tree *Prunus amygdalus* or *dulcis*

Mythology

Agdistis was an ancient Phrygian hermaphroditic deity, born from the earth mother after she was accidentally impregnated by the sleeping sky god. Pausanias translated the myth into Greek, naming the sky god Zeus. The gods castrated the hermaphrodite, who they were afraid of and his male organ fell onto the ground where it grew into an almond tree. No longer a hermaphrodite, Agdistis became the goddess Kybele. When the almonds were ripe, Nana, a Naiad-nymph of the river Saggarios, sat under the tree. One of the almonds fell from the tree and impregnated her. She gave birth to a boy, Attis, who she left on the mountainside to die. As is usual in such stories he was rescued by an animal, in this case, a goat and he grew up to become the consort of Kybele.

Botanical Description

The almond is a dense, rounded, deciduous tree or a large shrub, 4-9 m tall, with many branches, spreading out as wide as it is high. Two or more almond trees are needed for pollination to occur, usually by bees. Almond trees cover themselves with five-petaled, light pink to white flowers in early spring before the leaves appear. The flowers stick out from twigs or short side branches, then after pollination the green, oblong almond fruit develops over the next 7-8 months. The hull splits open to reveal the nut inside. Almond trees have little, green, oblong, pointed leaves with serrated edges.

Healing Properties of Almonds

Almonds help to maintain a healthy cardiovascular system, lower the risk of heart disease, help athletes to increase their performance and provide the body with many important vitamins and minerals.

Chemical constituents

Almonds contain vitamins: E, thiamin, riboflavin, niacin, pantothenic acid, B6 and folate; minerals: calcium, iron, magnesium, phosphorus, potassium, sodium, zinc, copper and manganese; proteins, amino acids, phenolic compounds and unsaturated fats.

Research

According to Abdulla in 2017 Unani medical practitioners consider that almond is an important food and medicine and use it to prevent and treat disease, both the body and brain. They use it to treat anaemia, loss of memory, insomnia, headache, cough and many other conditions.

In 2007 Sultana found that almond oil protected mice from the damaging effects of ultraviolet light. Human skin suffers from the harmful effects of sunlight, so it would be interesting to see whether almond oil could protect it. Long term studies would need to be carried out and it is unlikely that this will happen. However, people have been using almond oil on their skin without harmful side effects for some considerable time, as well as, of course, eating almonds.

Doctors have been advising people to cut down on saturated fat in order to reduce the risk of heart disease. But low-fat diets also lower high density lipoprotein cholesterol. We need cholesterol, which is made by our livers. It is a sterol and a structural component of all cell membranes, especially nerve and brain tissue. It's also a precursor of hormones and vitamins produced by the body. Lipoproteins transport it in the blood between the organs of the body. Cholesterol is not the problem. The problem is the type of lipoprotein, whether high density or low density. Low density lipoproteins are associated with atherosclerosis and heart disease. High density lipoproteins are not. In 2017 Berryman and team in the US found that 43 grams of almonds per day prevented levels of high-density lipoprotein cholesterol from decreasing in normal weight patients on a low cholesterol diet.

In 2007 Li and his team in China found that eating almonds protected smokers from the harmful effects of tobacco smoke. Cigarette smoke causes free radicals to form in the body of the smoker. Free radicals can damage the DNA inside the nucleus of cells, leading to Parkinson's disease, multiple sclerosis, Alzheimers and/or cancer. According to Li the antioxidants in almonds help to neutralise these free radicals.

In 2008 the US Food and Drug Administration authorised a claim that at least 42 grams of nuts per serving would reduce the risk of coronary heart disease. But nut consumption only reduces low density lipoprotein cholesterol by 5 percent. Yet studies have found that nut consumption lowers coronary heart disease risk by 30 percent. Phenolic compounds in the skins of almonds may partly be responsible for protecting the heart. In 2002 Sang isolated nine phenolic compounds from almond skins, including catechin and vanillic acid. In 2006 Wijeratne found that the skins of almonds were powerfully antioxidant. The Vitamin E in almonds is also a powerful antioxidant and these antioxidants probably protect the heart.

Chronic overeating can lead to chronic high levels of insulin. Insulin stimulates cells in the liver to restore glycogen and turn excess sugar into fatty acids. When there is too much insulin in the blood stream the body stops breaking down fat in tissue to use as energy and uses sugar, fatty acids and proteins in the blood as energy. When insulin levels remain high, cells become resistant to insulin signalling and glucose, fatty acids and cholesterol build up in the blood stream, causing cardiovascular disease, endocrine disorders and type 2 diabetes. So, in 2008 Jenkins and his team gave 70-75 grams of raw, un-blanched almonds per day to 27 overweight subjects who were following a low-fat diet. They found that their insulin levels fell.

Since inflammation plays a role in developing heart disease and some cancers, in 2009 Rajaram and team gave almonds to patients and measured indicators of inflammation in their blood, compared to the same indicators in the blood of a control group who didn't eat the almonds. They found that eating 68 almonds per 2,000 kilograms consumed lowered the amount of inflammation indicators in their blood. The results were interesting, since they add to the evidence that is accumulating that almond consumption might lower the risk of heart disease, but the study was small and further, bigger trials would be a good idea.

In 2014 Yi and team found that athletes who consumed almonds were able to cycle further and had better endurance than a group who didn't eat any almonds. Almonds contain the phenolic compounds, quercetin and arginine, which stimulate cells to generate more mitochondria, the energy producing organelles in the body's cells. Quercetin and arginine also stimulate oxygen delivery to muscle, so they suggested that almond consumption may help the body to use carbohydrates and oxygen more efficiently.

Almonds may be beneficial for people suffering from osteoporosis since they contain calcium, phosphorus and magnesium, all important minerals for the formation of bone.

In the US almonds are pasteurised. This may change the chemical structure of the oil in them. One of the pasteurisation methods involves chemical propylene oxide (once an additive to racing car fuel), a reactive genotoxic agent which may be carcinogenic. There is no law in the US that the type of pasteurisation technique should be shown on the labels of packaged almonds. For the full health benefits, almonds should be eaten raw, unpasteurised, in their skins and they should always be eaten fresh. The beneficial oils in almonds deteriorate over time, especially in a warm environment.

Contraindications

Some people are allergic to almonds.

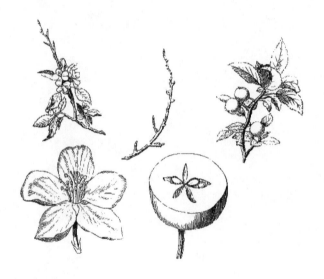

Apple tree *Malus domestica*

Mythology

When we slice open an apple crosswise, we reveal a pentagram of five pips, while sliced lengthwise we reveal a heart, both symbols of the goddess Aphrodite, divine guardian of harmonic order and proportion. Apparently when students began their first day at the Pythagorean mystery schools, they were each handed an apple sliced in half and asked to meditate upon it. The pentagram is a golden figure and we are reminded of it in the Homeric hymn to Aphrodite, the copper-haired goddess.

According to Apollodurus, the earth goddess Gaia produced the first sacred apple tree and gave it to the goddess Hera as a wedding present. The Ladon dragon twisted and twined, serpent-like around the tree in the Garden of the Hesperides, guarding the golden apples. Hera was a jealous goddess who tormented the illegitimate offspring of her unfaithful husband, Zeus. One of these was Hercules, who she sent to kill the Ladon dragon, in the hopes that he would not survive. But Hercules succeeded in killing the dragon, much to Hera's annoyance.

Apollodorus also tells the story of the three goddesses and the golden apple. Zeus held a banquet to celebrate the marriage of Peleus and Thetis. Eris, Goddess of discord, was not invited but she gatecrashed and threw a golden apple into the ceremony with an inscription on it saying "for the most beautiful." Hera, Athena and Aphrodite went to Zeus to claim the apple but Zeus handed the decision over to Paris. Hera offered to make Paris king of Europe and Asia Minor, Athena offered him wisdom and skill in battle and Aphrodite offered to make Helen of Troy fall in love with him, despite the fact that she was married to King Menelaus. Foolish Paris chose Aphrodite, which resulted in the Trojan war and the destruction of both Troy and Paris.

Apollodorus, Hesiod and Ovid all tell the story of Atalanta and the golden apples. Atalanta was a swift-footed huntress who offered to marry anyone who could outrun her, with the proviso that she would kill all those who she overtook with her spear. Milanion, knowing how fast she was, went to Aphrodite to ask for help. She gave him three golden apples from the garden of the Hesperides, which he dropped at strategic intervals. Atalanta stopped to pick them up, lost the race and married him. Overcome with passion, the two made love in the shrine of the Goddess Cybele. The gods and goddesses were angry and turned the pair into lions.

The *epimelides* were nymphs whose name derived from *epi* - protector and *melon* - sheep or apple tree. Thus, the *epimelides* were protectors of flocks and apple orchards. The apple, an important fruit in ancient Greece, was associated with love and marriage.

Botanical Description

Apple trees, which originated in central Asia, can grow to a considerable height and put out grey young stems and branches in the early spring. Later in spring they cover themselves in white or pink blossoms up to 5 cm wide. Then after pollination and the petals have fallen like a shower of snow, the trees produce elliptic ovate leaves with hairy undersides about 15 cm long.

Healing Properties of Apple

The old saying "an apple a day keeps the doctor away" is sound advice. Apples, eaten raw and whole, including the skin, help to protect the blood vessels from the build-up of fatty deposits, help to prevent heart disease, cancer, diabetes, asthma and bronchial hypersensitivity. It is important to avoid pesticides by eating organic apples.

Chemical constituents

According to Boyer and Liu in 2004 apples are a rich source of phytochemicals, such as flavonoids, isoflavonoids and phenolic acids, all of which are strong antioxidants. Other antioxidant compounds in apples include various quercetin compounds, catechin, epicatechin, procyanidin, cyanidin-3-galactoside, coumaric acid, chlorogenic acid, gallic acid and phloridzin. Apple peel contains procyanidins, catechin, epicatechin, chlorogenic acid, phloridzin and quercetin conjugates. Quercetin conjugates are only in the peel. Quercetin is a strong antioxidant and inhibits cancer cell growth *in vitro*. Different varieties of apples contain different amounts of each compound. Apples do not deteriorate during storage but apple juice loses most of its important phytochemicals.

Research

Apple peel contains more antioxidant compounds, more flavonoids and can stop cancer cells from growing better than apple flesh, according to Eberhardt in 2000. De Silva and team found that epicatechin and catechin are powerful antioxidants and inhibit low density lipoprotein (bad fats) from becoming oxidised *in vitro*. When low density lipoproteins become oxidised, they can stick to the walls of blood vessels and can cause atheroschlerosis (hardening and thickening of the arteries.) Clorogenic acid is a strong free radical scavenger.

According to Hertog in 1993, in Finland people consume most of their dietary flavonoids from apples and onions. In 2002 Knekt and his team carried out a study of about 10,000 people, in Finland. They found that those who consumed more flavonoids were less likely to die from heart disease, cancer or diabetes. The people who ate apples consumed high levels of quercetin which was in the apple peel and the researchers concluded that the quercetin protected them from type 2 diabetes. In the same study eating apples and oranges protected the participants from asthma. The researchers concluded that quercetin, hesperidin and naringenin were responsible for the asthma protective effect.

In 2003 Breinholt found that quercetin alone did not prevent fats from oxidising when he fed it to rats, suggesting that it is not the only compound responsible for apple's ability to prevent fats from oxidising. But since apple peel contains numerous other antioxidant compounds, they concluded that the combination of the different compounds and possible interaction between them probably adds up to an antioxidant effect. This may well protect the blood vessels and the heart from damage from cholesterol. In 2001 Aprikian and team found that when they fed apples to rats, they excreted more cholesterol. They also had less cholesterol and high-density lipoprotein in their blood.

When compared to many other fruits in the US, apples had the second highest level of antioxidant activity and the second highest concentration of phenolic compounds, more than pears or peaches, according to Sun in 2002.

In 2000 Feskanich and team carried out an epidemiological study and found that people who regularly ate apples had a reduced risk of some cancers, especially lung cancer. In 2003 Woods and team carried out a study involving 1,600 adults in Australia. They found that eating apples and pears protected people from asthma and bronchial hypersensitivity. Similarly, in 2001 in the UK Shaheen and team found that adults who ate apples tended to suffer fewer asthma attacks.

In 2003 de Oliviera carried out a study in Brazil on middle aged overweight women suffering from high cholesterol. They found that the women who ate apples and pears lost weight.

In 2003 Wolfe and her team found that apple peel had potent antioxidant activity and stopped liver cancer and colon cancer cells from growing *in vitro*. Vitamin C in apples contributes less than 0.4% of the antioxidant activity. Also, in 2003 Aprikian found that combined apple pectin and apple phenolic compounds lowered cholesterol in the liver and the blood. This combination also lowered the absorption of triglycerides and cholesterol far better than either apple pectin alone or apple phenolics alone. The pectin is in the apple flesh and most of the phenolic compounds are in the skin. So, we should always eat the whole apple including the skin, raw for maximum benefit.

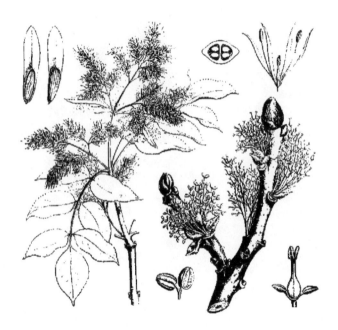

Ash manna *Fraxinus ornus*

Mythology

Hesiod relates how Kronos cut off the genitals of Ouranos, his father, and flung them onto Gaia, the earth. The first ash tree, together with the ash tree *meliae* (nymphs,) sprang from the spilt blood. *Meli*, or manna, sky-fallen juice of the stars, drips from the tree in the summer. The *meliai* nursed their sons on the sweet manna and armed them with ash wood spears. Ida and Adrasteia, two *meliai*, nursed the baby Zeus on ash tree manna and milk from the goat Amaltheia, on the island of Crete. Hesiod describes in his Theogony how the *meliai* were born together with the *erinyes* and the *gigantes*, who all wanted to avenge Ouranos. Together they eventually brought about the downfall of Kronos.

Homer's Iliad speaks of Ares, chief of the fierce Abantes, ravenous spear men, with long hair flowing down their backs. Ares was the father of the Amazons, fierce horsewomen, whose spears, made from the stem of the young ash, could pierce the corselets of their enemies.

Again, in the Iliad, Homer tells how Chiron made a spear from an ash tree growing on Mount Pelion for Peleus, who gave the spear to his son Achilles. Achilles and Asteropaeus, commander of the men of Paeonia, stood facing each other in the river, brandishing their spears and hurling insults at each other, until Asteropaeus threw spears from both hands simultaneously. One spear hit Achilles' shield which did not break while the other spear grazed Achilles' right forearm and landed in the ground. Achilles let fly his straight-flying ash spear at Asteropaeus but he missed and the spear plunged into the high river bank and stuck there. Asteropaeus tried to pull the spear out of the bank and as he struggled with it, Achilles killed him with his sword.

Botanical Description

The manna ash, called *melia* in Greek, is a small, round-headed deciduous tree which grows up to 15 m, with deep green, pointed oval leaves. In the Spring it covers itself with loose, branching clusters of fragrant creamy-white flowers. In the Summer the bark and leaves secrete a sweet sap known as manna, a sugary substance which people used to harvest up until the early part of the twentieth century, to sell it in the market. The word for both honey and manna is *meli* in Greek, for the ancients thought manna and honey were closely related.

In Greece people used to make a vertical series of oblique incisions in the trunk from July to the end of September. A whitish glutinous liquid exuded from the cuts, hardened and was harvested. After nine years the tree was exhausted so people cut it down, leaving one shoot to grow back. It took 4-5 years before this shoot was productive. Manna ash trees could produce about 6 kg of high-quality manna and 80 kg of assorted manna per hectare, according to Hendrick in 1972.

In the 19th century manna was exported to the United States for use as a pharmaceutical product. According to The Dispensatory of the United States of America, and according to Hill in 1952, manna from the manna ash was used as a mild laxative. According to Uphof in 1959, it is a tonic, especially useful for children and pregnant women. Modern editions of the Dispensatory simply discuss ash tree manna's active component "mannitol" without mention of ash trees. According to Brown in 1995, it was used as a sugar-free sweetener and anti-caking agent.

Healing Properties of manna ash bark and leaves

Fraxinus bark and leaves are wound healing, anti-fever, anti-rheumatic and anti-inflammatory. Traditionally the leaves are used to treat arthritic and rheumatic pain, myalgia and fever.

Chemical constituents

In 2002 Kostova isolated hydroxy-coumarins, secoiridoids, phenylethanoids, flavonoids and lignans from the bark, flowers and leaves.

Research

2002 Kostova reviewed the research that was carried out on *Fraxinus ornus*. She found that the bark was anti-microbial, anti-inflammatory, immuno-modulatory, skin-regenerating, antioxidant, anti-viral and it would prevent photo-dynamic damage. She demonstrated that extract of the stem bark and its main constituent esculin were non-toxic, anti-bacterial and prevented sun damage, especially when they contained hydroxy-coumarins. The hydroxy-coumarins prevented sun damage and were anti-microbial and antioxidant. She found that the extract and esculin were anti-inflammatory and speeded up the wound healing process in mice. But there have not been any clinical trials with manna ash, so although it is used traditionally in Greece, I cannot recommend anyone using the bark.

Unfortunately, the habit of collecting manna from the tree seems to have ceased, probably because an awful lot of trees are needed to produce a very small amount of manna. It is, nevertheless, an interesting tree.

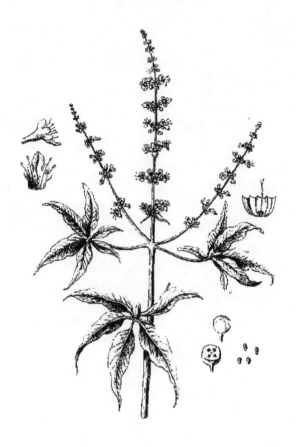

Chaste tree *Vitex agnus castus*

Mythology

Vitex agnus castus has been a symbol of chastity since ancient times: the vestal virgins in Rome once carried chaste tree twigs to symbolise their chastity, and chaste tree blossoms are still used ceremonially today in Italian monasteries to symbolise the celibacy of monastic life.

Pausanias mentions that the Goddess Hera was born and nursed under a *lygos* tree (*Vitex Agnus-castus*, the chaste-tree) on the island of Samos. The tree was sacred to Hera and associated with chastity. It was also sacred to Hestia, whose virgin priestesses carried chaste-tree stems; to Artemis, whose Spartan statue was bound in its stems; and to Demeter. People built a large temple and sanctuary in honour of Hera on the island and held an annual festival at which the image of Hera was bound with *lygos* branches and taken down to the sea to be washed. Apparently, according to Pausanias, there was still a chaste tree in the sanctuary in Roman times, although he did not visit Samos.

Hermes was the son of Zeus and the shy, nymph Maia, who lived in a cave where she bore their son. Hermes climbed out of his crib on the first day of his life, and stole fifty of Apollo's cattle.

Somehow, he managed to point their hoofs in the opposite direction from which he drove them. An old shepherd saw the baby Hermes driving cattle. When he climbed back into his crib his mother scolded him.

"Go and report to your father Zeus," she said angrily.

Zeus told Apollo, who confronted Hermes.

"How could I have stolen the cattle?" Hermes said innocently, "I'm a one-day old baby."

"Take us to where the cattle are hidden," Zeus demanded.

So, Zeus, Apollo and Hermes set off to find the cattle. When Apollo saw his cattle, he thought to himself,

"If Hermes is strong enough to drive my cattle on the first day of his life, he'll be a real danger when he grows up."

So, he tied him with chaste-tree binding, but the bands fell off him and began growing to cover all the wild-roving cattle. Hermes gave Apollo a lyre and they agreed that cattle for a lyre was a fair exchange.

According to Pausanius, Hermes did not steal the god's cattle, but he separated them, bound them with the chaste tree, and bred them. He increased their fertility by feeding the chaste tree to cows and other female livestock, since we have modern evidence that it aids menstrual problems and increases fertility. He may have fed it to the bulls that he did not want to breed. Thus, Hermes the god, taught humans how to care for animals by breeding and became the father of animal husbandry. This myth is about the period of time in which people began to domesticate animals.

Galen said:

"The fruit of the chaste tree... keeps in check sexual impulses — both the roasted and the un-roasted fruit do so — and the leaves and flowers of the shrub can do this same thing, so that it is trusted to effect chastity, not only when it is eaten and drunk but also when it is strewn underneath as bedding... it not only does not spur them (sexual appetites) on but also by nature suppresses them."

Pliny said that the chaste tree inhibits sexual desire.

Thesmophoria was an annual festival, dedicated to Demeter, in which Greek women went on a retreat for three to ten days in the late Autumn. On the second day the women fasted for the day and slept that night on a bed of chaste tree twigs and leaves. Pliny wrote:

"The Greeks call it lygos, sometimes agnos, because the Athenian matrons, preserving their chastity at the Thesmophoria, strew their beds with its leaves."

Heinrich von Staden, who studied the *Thesmophoria* and the chaste tree, confirms that the women slept on the twigs, leaves and bark of the chaste tree, abstaining from food and sexual activity. (This must have been incredibly uncomfortable!) Von Staden saw its meaning as

"...not only a regression into pre-cultural wildness, but also a new beginning, at the very inception both of culture and of human life."

Dioscorides wrote,

"It [chaste tree] draws down milk and it brings on the menses when a quantity of one drachma is drunk with wine; but it also slackens the organ of generation, and it affects the head inducing deep sleep. The decoction of the plant itself and of its fruit helps in sitz baths for conditions and inflammations of the uterus."

Botanical Description

Vitex agnus-castus, which belongs to the verbena family, the *Verbenaceae,* is an aromatic, small deciduous tree, 3-5 m high or a large bush. It has 5-7 lobed leaves, each lobe of which is slender and pointed. The leaves, which grow opposite each other are dark green above, grey underneath and covered in a soft felt. It forms small violet, blue, pink or white flowers in dense, apical flower heads. The *Vitex agnus-castus* fruit, sometimes called chaste-berry, is brown, half covered by sage green calyx, with 4 seeds and about the size of a peppercorn.

Healing Properties

Vitex agnus-castus is a woman's herb, used to alleviate PMS and a more severe form called premenstrual dysphoric disorder. It is used for reducing and preventing breast pain, for balancing female hormones, for treating and preventing female acne, and for alleviating menopausal symptoms. It was possibly used to decrease men's libido during the middle ages according to Tesch in 2003.

Chemical constituents

Vitex agnus castus fruit contains essentials oils, flavonoids and oestrogen-like compounds, such as apigenin. Compounds in the essential oils include diterpenes, 4-terpinol, alpha pinene, beta phellandrene, sabinene, beta caryophyllene, beta farnesine and spathulenol and clerodadienols which stimulate the pituitary gland to produce dopamine. Flavonoids include orientin, zyloside, vitexin and isovitexin.

Research

There has been an enormous amount of interest in the healing properties of *Vitex agnus castus* and numerous scientists have carried out research, especially clinical trials, which have demonstrated that Chaste tree berries are effective at rebalancing the female hormone system. I am not going to attempt to cover all the research since my readers would fall asleep before I reached the end of it, but I will mention a few clinical trials, which usually used a pharmaceutical preparation based on extract of *Vitex*. Herbalists in Britain however, tend to use tinctures of *Vitex*, as described by Kerry Hughs in 2006. She reported on the results of a questionnaire that 153 members of the National Institute of British Medical Herbalists filled in, regarding the use of *Vitex agnus castus*. 94% of the herbalists used it to treat PMS, 86% used it to treat menopausal symptoms, 89% used it to treat infertility and 79% used it to treat female acne. 98% of the respondents said that *Vitex* was very effective for rebalancing female hormone levels.

Premenstrual symptoms may be related to high levels of prolactin, a hormone which stimulates the production of breast milk and regulates the menstrual cycle, among many other things. Dopamine, a brain chemical, inhibits the pituitary gland from releasing prolactin. *Vitex agnus castus* fruit contains diterpenes, which stimulate the pituitary gland to produce dopamine, which in turn reduces prolactin, which improves premenstrual symptoms. In 2019 Csupor found that women taking part in a clinical trial with *Vitex agnus castus* extracts were 2.5 times more likely to find that their symptoms were reduced, compared to those taking a placebo. Some of the women said that their symptoms disappeared. In 2004 Wuttke found that a clinical trial with a German chaste tree product: Mastodynon (Bionorica AG Neumarkt) resulted in significantly less breast pain and lower prolactin levels in patients with premenstrual breast pain. Diterpene compounds called clerodadienols in the extract were responsible for the dopamine stimulating effect.

Vitex agnus castus fruits also contain oestrogen-like compounds, such as apigenin, that may help alleviate menopausal symptoms. Some women experience breast tenderness, menorrhagia, migraine, nausea and/or shorter cycle length, which are caused by too much oestrogen. Alternatively, they may suffer vasomotor symptoms, and vaginal dryness, which are caused by lack of oestrogen. These symptoms often alternate, along with mood swings, dysfunctional uterine bleeding and hot flashes during the menopausal transition. In 2009 Van Die found that most of the herbal formulations used to treat menopausal symptoms contained several different herbs, including *Vitex agnus castus*. The menopause herbal formulation Phyto-Female Complex (SupHerb; Netanya, Israel), which contains *Vitex agnus castus* berries, prevented menopausal hot flashes and night sweats significantly better than placebo in 50 healthy peri- and post-menopausal women.

In 2014 Eftekhari and team carried out a clinical trial in Iran, giving *Vitex agnus castus* and magnesium to women suffering from bone fractures. 64 women aged 24-45 took part. The researchers divided the women into 4 groups and gave *Vitex* extract and magnesium to one group, *Vitex* extract and placebo to a second group, magnesium and placebo to a third group and both placebos to the 4th group. At the end of the trial the bones of the women who had been taking the *Vitex* extract and magnesium together were healing faster than the other groups. This was a small trial but the results suggest that *Vitex agnus castus* may speed up bone healing in younger women. More research and bigger trials are needed to confirm these interesting results.

In 1996 Snow found that *Vitex agnus castus* acts directly on the pituitary gland, increasing luteinizing hormone (LH) production and inhibiting the release of follicle stimulating hormone (FSH). As already mentioned, it also inhibits prolactin secretion. It can be used to treat women who do not have enough corpus luteum, which causes symptoms such as: excessively long or heavy menses, more frequent than normal menstrual cycles, scanty or painful or abnormally heavy or long menstruation, the absence of menstruation, lack of ovulation or infertility. It can also be used for insufficient lactation, too much prolactin in the blood, breast pain, and premenstrual acne.

In 2019 Jazani reviewed the clinical studies with herbal medicine on polycystic ovary syndrome. They found that a wide spectrum of herbs can be used to improve polycystic ovary syndrome, including *Vitex agnus castus*. In 2003 Dericks-Tan carried out a clinical trial giving a German *Agnus castus* extract product or placebo to healthy men for fourteen days. They found that the men who took the *Agnus castus* product had increased levels of melatonin and fell asleep more quickly.

Contraindications

People taking dopamine agonists or antagonists should not take *Vitex agnus castus*. Nor should pregnant or breast-feeding women.

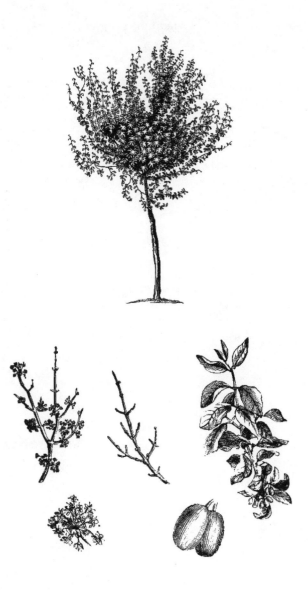

Cherry tree Cornelian *Cornus mas*

Mythology

The mythology surrounding the cornelian cherry (*kraneiai*) is somewhat unclear, though the ancients living in Greece before the era of written myth do appear to have eaten the fruit. It may have grown in Apollo's precinct on Mount Ida, until the Greeks cut it down, subsequently offering sacrifices to propitiate the God, who they now called *Karneios* (rather than *Kraneios*). According to Charles M. Skinner, a cornelian cherry sprang from the grave of Polydorus, who was slain by Polymnestor. Apparently, it dripped blood when Aeneas tried to pull its branches from its trunk. But according to Virgil that tree was a myrtle. According to Athenaeus, Kraneia, the nymph of the cornelian cherry tree was one of the eight hamadryad daughters of the forest-spirit Oxylos and the nymph Hamadryas, who lived on Mount Oita in Northern Greece.

Botanical Description

Cornelian cherry is not really a cherry at all, but a member of the dogwood family, the Cornaceae. It can grow up to a maximum 12 m, either as a large shrub or an oval-headed tree, usually branching near the ground. In full sun the branches are largely upright, whereas in shade the branches spread wide to catch the limited light. The flowers are tiny with 4 yellow petals and grow in clusters of 10-25, early in the spring before the leaves appear. The fruits are oblong, red, 2 cm long, 1.5 cm diameter, edible and contain a single seed. The satiny green oval leaves grow opposite each other with leaf veins growing almost out to the edges of the leaves then joining together to follow the leaf margins in parallel. Bright red fruits ripen in late summer.

Healing Properties of *Cornus mas*

Cornelian cherry has anti-microbial, anti-parasitic, anti-inflammatory, antioxidant and anti-cancer properties, as well as protecting liver, kidney and cardiovascular system. The fruits are used in traditional medicine to treat a wide variety of diseases, including diarrhoea, inflammatory bowel disease, fever, type 2 diabetes and bleeding.

Chemical constituents

Scientists have identified over 100 different compounds from *Cornus mas*, including anthocyanins, flavonoids and iridoids, such as logic acid, loganin, sweroside and cornuside. The flavonoids and anthocyanidins in the fruits are powerfully antioxidant. The fruit also contains fructose, glucose and reducing sugars, potassium, calcium, sodium, iron, zinc, manganese, and copper. Cornelian cherry juice contains high levels of calcium, ten times higher (323 mg/L) than other juices.

Research

Most of the research into the healing properties of *Cornus mas* has been carried out in the laboratory. Several researchers, including Dinda and Hosseinpour-Jaghdani in 2016 and in 2017 have reviewed the research into its therapeutic properties. Extracts of the fruits and other parts of the plant are anti-bacterial, anti-fungal, anti-diabetic, protect the blood vessels from fatty deposits, protect the liver and kidneys *in vitro*. In 2013 Deng and team found that the Cornelian cherry fruit compounds: loganin, sweroside, and cornuside, reduced the amount of DNA damage *in vivo*. Several different scientists including Asquary in 2014, have demonstrated that *Cornus mas* extracts lower blood sugar and fats in various animal models. Also, in 2014, Alavian demonstrated that extracts of *Cornus mas* fruits protected the liver of rats from damage. In 2010 Petridis found that *Cornus mas* fruits were highly antioxidant *in vitro*.

The research suggests that Cornelian cherry fruits and leaves could possibly be used to treat diabetes, obesity, atherosclerosis, skin diseases, gastrointestinal and rheumatic symptoms. There have been a few clinical trials, including one by Soltani and team evaluating the effects of *Cornus mas* on patients with type 2 diabetes. Soltani gave 2 capsules of *Cornus mas* extract, each containing 150 mg of anthocyanin, twice a day to 30 patients and placebo to the remaining 30. After 6 weeks the group taking the *Cornus mas* had significantly more insulin and less sugar in their blood than the control group, which suggests that the Cornelian cherry fruits may be effective for controlling type 2 diabetes. Of course, this was a small trial.

In 2013 Asgary and team carried out a clinical trial with 40 children and adolescents suffering from abnormal levels of blood fats. They gave 50g of *Cornus mas* twice a day to half the group. After 6 weeks they found that the children who had been taking the *Cornus mas* extract had lower levels of cholesterol, low density lipoprotein, triglycerides and less vascular inflammation than the group who took the placebo. This was a small trial but the results were interesting.

More research and especially clinical trials are needed to find out how the extracts, as well as the active compounds work, which conditions the Cornelian cherry could help and what the effective dosage should be. But people have been using the fruits as medicine for centuries without any apparent ill effect. In Britain we can grow the Cornelian cherry tree but summers are seldom hot enough to produce a ripe crop of fruit, but in Greece people traditionally make the fruits into jam.

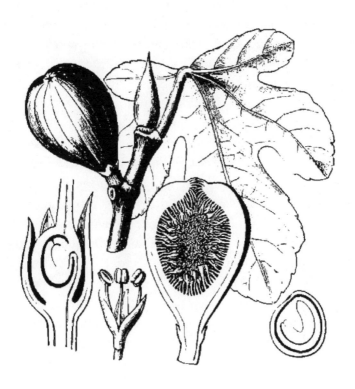

Fig tree *Ficus carica*

There are about 750 species of fig, according to Lansky in 2011. *Ficus carica*, wild fig, is native to Iran, Armenia, Azerbaijan, Georgia, Turkey, Kyrgyzstan Tajikistan, Turkmenistan and Uzbekistan. Figs are one of the most important wild edible plants used traditionally in Turkey; and Turkey is the world's leading producer of figs. People have been eating figs and using them as medicine since prehistoric times and the earliest evidence comes from Neolithic sites from the Jordan Valley about 10,000-8,000 BCE, according to Fuller in 2019.

Ripe dried figs, as well as the root and the leaves, are used in native medicine to treat colic, indigestion, loss of appetite, sore throats, coughs and bronchial symptoms, according to Penelope in 1997. In 2005 Brussel found that in Greek folk medicine eating large quantities of figs is thought to expel intestinal worms. People use the fruit's juice mixed with honey for haemorrhage and apply the fruit paste to swelling tumours and inflammation. The fig leaves are used to treat diabetes, high cholesterol, eczema, psoriasis and vitiligo. In Europe fig powder is authorised for use as a skin-conditioning component in cosmetic products.

Mythology

According to Athenaeus, Sykeus the Titan waged war on the gods so Zeus chased him to Cilicia, where he hid in the bosom of his mother, Gaia, who transformed him into a fig tree. The Hamadryad nymph of the fig tree was called Hamadryas Syke.

According to Pausanias, as Demeter roamed the earth, searching for her daughter, Kore, she came to Eleusis in Attica, where she stopped at the house of Phytalus who welcomed her and gave her a drink. To thank him she created a fig tree, which resulted in the fig tree being sacred to Demeter, as well as to

Dionysos. Pliny listed 29 varieties, together with information on the locations where each was grown, according to Condit in 1955.

Botanical Description

Figs depend on the female fig wasp for pollination. The fig tree is gynodioecious (having female flowers on one tree and hermaphrodite flowers on another) and functionally dioecious (male and female flowers occur on separate trees.) The female trees have long-styled female flowers that do not host wasp larvae. Male fig trees have short-styled female flowers that host wasp larvae but produce very few seeds. Figs from functionally male trees produce pollen and harbour wasps. When a wasp emerges from a fig cavity covered with pollen, it has about one day to find and enter a receptive fig.

Fig trees are rarely more than 6 m high with broad, rough, deciduous, deeply lobed leaves, though wild figs often have almost entire leaves. Figs grow in the axils of the leaves, singly and are unique, for they produce something which is neither a fruit nor a flower. Each fig is a hollow, fleshy receptacle with a multitude of flowers inside, which manage to ripen and produce seeds without ever being exposed to the light of day.

Healing Properties

Figs are nutritious, laxative, demulcent, antioxidant, anti-bacterial. They have a calming effect on irritable bowel syndrome. Strangely they do not cause blood sugar levels to rise.

Chemical constituents

Figs are an excellent source of phenolic compounds such as pro-anthocyanidins. They contain arabinose, beta-amyrins, beta-carotines, glycosides, sterols, according to Duke 1992, as well as alkaoilds, anthraquinones, coumarins, flavonoids, saponins tannins and terpenes.

The leaves contain volatile compounds such as aldehydes, alcohols, ketones, methyl salicylate and monoterpenes.

Research

Most of the research that has been carried out was with crude extracts of fig tree fruit and leaves in the laboratory, either *in vitro* or *in vivo*. In 2000 Canal found that the leaf extract lowers blood sugar, while in 2002 Richter found that figs stop bleeding. In 2006 Solomon found that *Ficus carica* fruit is antioxidant. In 2009 Jeong demonstrated that figs are anti-bacterial. In 2010 Patil found that fig leaves lowered the temperature of rats.

In 2013 Shukranul reviewed the chemistry, biological activities and traditional uses of Ficus carica. He found that extracts of different parts of the fig tree had anticancer effects, protected the liver, reduced blood sugar and blood fats and were anti-bacterial and anti-fungal. In 2008 Fulani found that extracts of fig relaxed isolated muscles of rabbit intestines in the laboratory. This could explain some of its medicinal uses in hyperactive gut disorders.

There have been a few clinical trials, mostly on small numbers of patients. In 2019 Atkinson carried out a small double-blind study on ten healthy adults who drank 4 test beverages containing 100, 200, 600 and 1,200 mg of fig extract. He found that postprandial blood glucose levels were reduced at the higher levels and insulin levels were reduced at all levels. In 2015 Sardari carried out a trial on 40 patients with multiple sclerosis who suffered from constipation. He gave half the patients 10g of fig paste and half the patients a placebo. He found that the patients who took the fig paste said that their symptoms improved. In 2017 Tofighi studied the effect of a fig and flaxseed combination on 15 patients suffering from constipation. All the patients said that their symptoms improved. In 2019 Pourmasoumi found that eating flixweed (*Descurainia sophia*) or figs caused significant improvement in irritable bowel syndrome symptoms in a randomised controlled trial with 150 patients with IBS. In 2016 Bahadori conducted a clinical investigation on the effects of olive oil and an olive fruit and fig mixture on 56 patients suffering from rheumatoid arthritis. Patients either received methotrexate alone, or together with fig/olive mixture. Those who took the fig/olive mixture together with the methotrexate said that their symptoms improved.

People have been eating figs since the dawn of time. They are nutritious and delicious and undoubtedly have many medicinal properties.

Contraindications

Eating too many figs they can cause flatulence, pain in the bowels and diarrhoea.

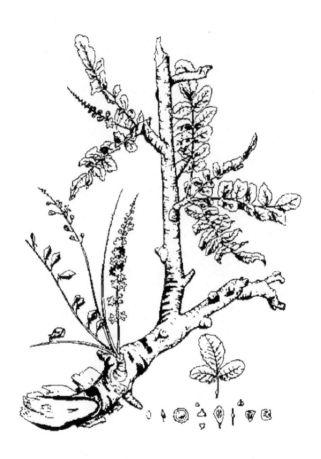

Frankincense tree *Boswellia carterii*

In many parts of the world people believe that breathing the scent which is released from the burning resin connects them to the spiritual world and calls forth the angels, which may explain why it is used in religious ceremonies. The smoke that rises carries prayers and offerings to Heaven. Using it in meditation has a calming effect.

According to Shishodia in 2008, the history of Frankincense (*guggul* in Ayurveda) goes as far back as 1700 BCE. The *Sushruta Samhita*, an ancient Indian script on medicine and surgery, states that *guggul* when taken orally can cure internal tumours, malignant sores, obesity, liver dysfunction, intestinal worms, leucoderma, and oedema. Ayurvedic doctors also use it to prevent and treat inflammatory bowel disease, ulcers, arthritis, cardiovascular diseases, diabetes etc. People have been using gum resin extracts of Boswellia species traditionally in many parts of the world for centuries to treat various chronic inflammatory diseases, such as rheumatism, asthma, bronchitis, pancreatitis, earache, psoriasis and gastrointestinal disorders.

Mythology

According to Ovid there once was a Persian princess who was loved by the sun-god Helios. When her father learned of the affair, he buried her in the sand. Helios then transformed her body into the frankincense tree and ever since then the frankincense tree has been sacred to Helios.

Botanical Description

There are nineteen species of *Boswellia* trees, which grow in Arabia and north Africa, are shrubby and small, with flaking bark and small pinnate leaves directly attached to the twigs. They have no thorns. The flowers have 5 petals, with internal stamens that are disk-shaped in the centre. The fruits and seeds are similar to capsules, and when they are ripe they release 3-5-winged nutlets from the outer layer. These plant species are bisexual and can self-pollinate. The ancient Greeks imported the aromatic gum to use as incense in religious ceremonies.

Unfortunately, in 2019 Frans Bongers discovered that *Boswellia* trees are in danger. He relates how the young trees are being prevented from growing by grazing cattle and frequent fires. The old trees are gradually dying off.

Healing Properties

Frankincense reduces anxiety, stimulates the immune system, diminishes signs of ageing, anxiety/depression and memory loss, improves brain function in Alzheimer's disease, helps ageing skin and flagging libido. It is anti-inflammatory and will help to alleviate the symptoms of Crohn's disease and ulcerative colitis. Used externally it helps to alleviate the pain of rheumatoid arthritis. It is antiseptic and decongestant so good for sore throats and infections of the broncho-pulmonary system, such as bronchitis.

Chemical constituents

The resinous part of *Boswellia serrata* contains monoterpenes, diterpenes, triterpenes, tetracyclic triterpenic acids and four major pentacyclic triterpenic acids which inhibit the enzymes which cause inflammation; as well as a huge number of lignans and ketosterols, which contribute to its health benefits. The most famous compounds in frankincense are the boswellic acids.

Research

According to Pubmed; "google," there are 519 publications on *Boswellia* and 329 on boswellic acid. Numerous studies, both in the laboratory and with human subjects, confirm that extracts from the various *Boswellia* species could potentially be used to treat inflammation, cancer and ulcerative colitis.

When Singh carried out clinical trials with *Boswellia* gum-resin on patients with osteoarthritis, and rheumatoid arthritis in 1984, he found that it improved their symptoms. Several scientists, including Sing in 2012, found that *Boswellia serrata* extract was antioxidant and free radical scavenging *in vitro*. This could be due in part to the various phenolic compounds in *Boswellia* species. In 2006 Poeckel reviewed the biological actions of boswellic acids. They interfere with the signalling in various blood cells related with inflammation and tumour growth. In 2019 Doaee found that *Boswellia serrata* resin extracts protected the nerves of rats in an experimental model of Parkinson's disease.

Boswellia gum resin contains boswellic acids, which block leukotrienes, the cause of inflammation in ulcerative colitis. In 1997 Gupta carried out a clinical trial, giving *Boswellia serrata* gum resin to patients suffering from ulcerative colitis. 82 % of the patients who took *Boswellia serrata* gum resin found that their symptoms disappeared. In 2001 Gerhardt carried out a clinical trial with patients suffering from Crohn's disease, giving *Boswellia serrata* extract H 15 to half the patients and the pharmaceutical product, mesalazine to the other half. He found that both groups of patients' symptoms improved but the *Boswellia* extract caused fewer side effects.

Boswellia serrata is one of the most valued ancient herbs in Ayurveda. In 2011 Siddiqui reviewed the anti-inflammatory properties of *Boswellia serrata*, a species of *Boswellia* which grows in India, Northern Africa and the Middle East. Acetyl-11-keto-β-boswellic acid is the most potent inhibitor of 5-lipoxygenase, an enzyme which causes inflammation. Boswellic acids inhibit human leukocyte elastase (HLE) which is involved in emphysema. Since HLE stimulates mucus secretion it may be involved in cystic fibrosis, chronic bronchitis and acute respiratory distress syndrome, according to Rall in 1996. HLE starts to damage tissues and this triggers the inflammatory process. Boswellic acids are unique since they inhibit inflammation in 2 different ways.

How to Use

Put 4-5 small pieces of resin in a jar with 2 pints of boiled water and leave to steep overnight. Drink up to a cupful a day to treat ulcerative colitis.

Use the essential oil of frankincense diluted in a carrier, such as almond oil, to reduce the swelling caused by rheumatoid arthritis or osteoarthritis. Massage onto painful joints. Frankincense oil is sometimes called olibanum, has a sweet, woody scent and can be used in a diffuser to ease stress.

Dilute the essential oil with almond oil to use it for a whole-body massage. As you breathe it in or absorb it through your skin it sends messages to that part of the brain which influences emotions, lowering blood pressure and heart rate, calming anxiety and relaxing the whole body.

Be careful to buy frankincense essential oil from a reputable supplier and check the label for the Latin name, *Boswellia carterii* or *Boswellia sacra*. No other oil ingredients should be listed and if they are it indicates that the frankincense oil is diluted.

Contraindications

Some people are allergic to frankincense, so you should carry out a patch test before using it for aromatherapy. Pregnant and breast-feeding women should not use it.

Boswellia may interact with and decrease the effects of anti-inflammatory medications, such as ibuprofen, aspirin and other non-steroidal anti-inflammatory drugs. Talk to your doctor before using *Boswellia* products, especially if you're taking other medications to treat inflammation.

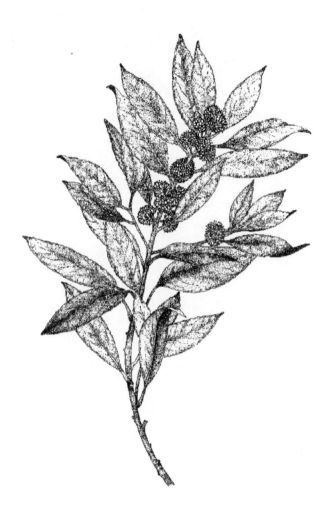

Laurel or Bay sweet *Laurus nobilis*

Mythology

According to Pausanias, Ovid and Hyginus, the god Apollo loved Daphne, an Arkadian Nymph. When he pursued her, she fled and transformed herself into a laurel tree to avoid being raped by him. The plant was ever after sacred to Apollo Daphnaios. Artemis had sacred laurel groves and was titled Daphnaia. The god and the victors of Apollo's Pythian Games were crowned with laurel wreaths.

Botanical Description

The laurel or sweet bay is a small tree, 2-15 m tall, with smooth bark which can be olive-green or reddish. The luxurious evergreen leaves with short stalks, grow alternately and are lanceolate with smooth, wavy margins. They are thick, smooth and shining dark green. Laurel produces male and female flowers, which are small, yellow, 4-lobed and grow in small clusters; the male has 8-12 stamens and the female 2-4 staminodes. The fruit is 1-1.5 cm, ovoid, and purplish black when ripe. It grows well under the shade of other trees. People cook with the aromatic leaves.

Healing properties

The leaves are antiseptic, aromatic, astringent, digestive, diuretic, anti-parasitic and stimulant. They relieve flatulence. If you boil them up and drink the resultant tea when suffering from a cold, they will bring out a sweat and rid the body of toxins, helping you to recover more quickly. In large doses they are emetic, emmenagogue and narcotic. They are used traditionally to treat bronchitis, influenza and to aid digestion. They have a tonic effect, stimulating the appetite and the secretion of digestive juices. The fruit is narcotic and people used it as an emmenagogue (a euphemism for a substance which produces an abortion).

Chemical constituents

Lauris nobilis contains sesquiterpene lactones such as 10-epigazaniolide, gazaniolide, spirafolide, costunolide, reynosin, santamarine; flavonoid glycosides and essential oil. The essential oil contains a multitude of compounds such as: cineole, α-terpinyl acetate, terpinene-4- ol, α-pinene, β- pinene, p-cymene and linalool acetate.

Research

In 2012 Patrakar reviewed the research that has been carried out on the chemistry and pharmacology of *Lauris nobilis*. Bay has wound healing, nerve-protective, antioxidant, anti-ulcer, anti-convulsant, anti-mutagenic, anti-viral, anti-cholinergic, anti-bacterial and anti-fungal properties.

In 1997 Afifi and team found that extracts of laurel seeds protected rats from ulcers. In 1998 Samejima and team isolated kaempferyl coumarate, an anti-mutagenic compound from bay laurel extract. In 2002 Sayyah and team demonstrated that essential oil from laurel leaf could protect rats from epileptic fits. They suggested that methyl-eugenol, eugenol and pinene might have been responsible for the anti-seizure effect. When they gave the rats big enough doses of the essential oil to stop the seizures, the animals were sedated and could hardly move. In 2003 Sayyah demonstrated that essential oil of *Laurus nobilis* leaf was analgesic and anti-inflammatory *in vivo*. In 2006 Nayak and team found that extracts of laurel were healing *in vivo*. In 2011 Ham found that laurel extracts protected the substantia nigra (a part of the brain that is affected by Parkinson's disease) of young adult rats. Two major compounds from the laurel extracts, costunolide and dehydrocostus lactone, were powerful nerve protectors.

In 2006 Elmastas and team demonstrated *in vitro* that laurel extracts were antioxidant and free radical scavenging. Also, in 2006 Ferreira and team found that the essential oil of laurel inhibited acetyl-cholinesterase *in vitro*. Acetyl-cholinesterase breaks down acetyl choline, a key neuro-transmitter which people suffering from Alzheimers tend to lack. So, laurel could, potentially, stop the breakdown of acetyl-choline and delay the onset of Alzheimers. Also, in 2006 Erler and team demonstrated that essential oils from the seeds and leaves of laurel *Laurus nobilis* repelled *Culex pipiens*, a common pest mosquito. In 2007 Corato and team demonstrated that extracts of laurel leaf were anti-fungal against the fungus *Botrytis cinerea* Pers. *in vitro*. In 2008 Loizzo and team demonstrated that essential oil of laurel leaf was anti-viral *in vitro*. In 2010 Ozcan and team found that an extract of laurel seed oil was anti-bacterial and antioxidant *in vitro*.

Many other scientists carried out research on bay leaf in the laboratory, but unfortunately no one has yet carried out any clinical trials to demonstrate that it could be used therapeutically. However, people have been cooking with bay leaves and using them as medicine for thousands of years.

It is easy to grow a small bay tree, either in a pot on a balcony or planted in your garden.

How to Use

Make a tea with 2 bay leaves and a pint of boiled water. Leave to steep for five minutes and drink to sooth a sore throat, cough, bronchitis. You can add ginger, honey, lemon.

Drink a bay leaf tea at bedtime to help you sleep.

Grind up 10-20 bay leaves and add them to your bath, to calm the mind and body. Their anti-inflammatory, antibacterial and anti-fatigue properties will relax aching muscles and joints.

When cooking with bay leaves be sure to remove them before eating.

Contraindications

Don't use bay leaves for at least two weeks before surgery because they might slow down the central nervous system too much during anaesthesia. People taking medications for high blood sugar should avoid bay leaf.

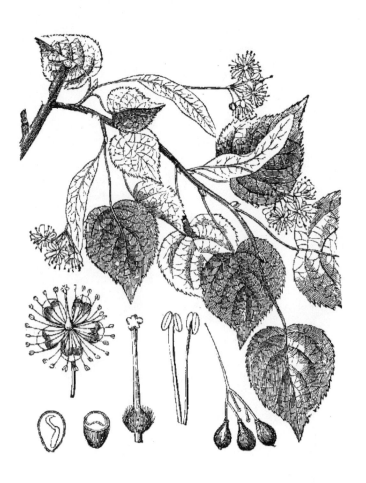

Lime or Linden, large-leafed *Tilia platyphyllos*

In China, according to Zhang in 2004, people use an infusion of *Tilia species* traditionally as sedatives and tranquillisers.

Mythology

According to Hyginus, Kronos loved the nymph, Philyra. When his wife Rhea interrupted their rendezvous, he transformed himself into a horse and fled. Alternate sources say that Philyra transformed herself into a horse to escape Kronos and he transformed himself into a stallion, chased after her and raped her. Both versions seem to agree that Philyra was later horrified by the sight of her new born half-horse baby (Chiron), who she abandoned. According to Hyginus she begged Zeus to change her form and he transformed her into a linden tree.

According to Ovid Philemon and Baukis were a pious couple who received the gods Zeus and Hermes hospitably when they were travelling amongst mankind in disguise. The gods destroyed those who had turned them away and rewarded the couple by making them priests of the temple and transforming them into a pair of entwined trees when they died: Baukis a linden, and Philemon an oak.

Botanical Description

Tilia platyphyllos is a narrowly domed tree which grows slowly, eventually reaching about 40m in height. The reddish-brown young stems later develop dark grey bark with fine fissures and furrows. The branches spread upwards at wide angles. The twigs are reddish-green and slightly hairy. The 6-9 cm leaves grow singly and alternately. They are mid to dark green above and below, with white downy hair on the underside, particularly along the veins, and are ovate to heart shaped, tapering to a sharp point. The leaf edges are sharply toothed and the base heart shaped with veins spread out from a central point along a midrib and 3-4 cm long stalks. The flowers, which are pollinated by bees, are small, fragrant, yellowish-white with 5 sepals, 5 petals and numerous stamens, and hang in drooping clusters in groups of 3-4 with whitish-green, leaf-like bracts. The fruit is a small, round, cream-coloured nutlet covered in a layer of matted woolly down, one centimetre or less diameter. It has a woody shell with 3-5 ridges. In Autumn the leaves turn yellow.

Healing Properties

Lime flower tea is anti-spasmodic, diaphoretic, expectorant, laxative, sedative and lowers blood pressure. People use lime flower and leaf tea traditionally to bring out a sweat during feverish colds, to treat infections, and to relieve nasal congestion, sore throat and cough. They also use the flowers to relieve mild symptoms of mental stress and anxiety-related indigestion, either as a tea or added to baths. People also use lime flower tea to treat nervous vomiting, cough, fever, infections, inflammation, high blood pressure, headache (particularly migraine), as a diuretic, anti-spasmodic (reduces smooth muscle spasm along the digestive tract) and sedative.

Chemical constituents

According to the European Medicines Agency in 2012 *Tilia* flowers contain:

caffeic, chlorogenic and p-coumaric acids; amino acids: alanine, cysteine, cystine, isoleucine, leucine, phenylalanine and serine; carbohydrates: mucilage polysaccharides (3%), which soothe and reduce inflammation, arabinose, galactose, rhamnose, with lesser amounts of glucose, mannose, and xylose; galacturonic and glucuronic acids; antioxidant flavonoids: kaempferol, quercetin, myricetin and their glycosides; volatile oil - (0.02% to 0.1%.) They contain alkanes, phenolic alcohols and esters, and terpenes: monoterpenes, including citral, citronellal, citronellol, eugenol, limonene, nerol, α-pinene and terpineol; and sesquiterpenes such as farnesol. Other constituents include an unspecified saponin, condensed tannin, tocopherol and volatile oils.

Research

Most of the research on lime flowers was carried out in the laboratory. In 1984 Guerin & Reveillere found that lime flower extracts were anti-fungal. In 1988 Taddei reported that the volatile oils of lime flowers were sedative and anti-spasmodic in mice. In 1994 Viola and team found that lime flower extracts were sedative in mice. In 1998 Blumenthal found that lime flower oil had a sedative effect on mice when they inhaled it. In 1999 Anesini and team demonstrated that lime flower extracts had sedative and anti-anxiety effect *in vitro*. In 2000 Blumenthal suggested that the diaphoretic activity of lime flowers may be due to quercetin, kaempherol and p-coumaric acid. In 2003 Nowak and team isolated tiliroside from *Tilia species* which kills human leukaemic cells *in vitro*. In 2010 Ranilla and team demonstrated that *Tilia platyphyllos* flowers were antioxidant *in vitro* and inhibited alpha glucosidase, an enzyme involved in high blood sugar and high blood pressure. They suggested that lime flowers may have a potential for the control of type 2 diabetes.

In 2010 scientists carried out a study for the World Health Organisation with 15 patients suffering from chronic catarrh. They found that patients who inhaled the steam from lime flowers in hot water improved more than control patients who inhaled steam without the lime flowers. This was a small study with no statistical analysis of the data, so further and larger randomised controlled clinical trials would need to be carried out in order to prove that lime flower inhalation is effective against catarrh. Apart from the above study there have been no clinical trials assessing the effects of lime flower. However, people have been using lime flowers for centuries as a tea or infusion and they are perfectly safe.

How to Use lime flowers

Make a herbal infusion with 1.5 g of dried lime flowers in 150 ml of boiling water and take 2–4 times daily to treat colds, coughs, catarrh. It will help to make a dry, irritating cough productive. Drink a lime flower infusion or put lime flowers in your bath when you are feeling anxious or having trouble falling asleep for their soothing, calming effect.

Contraindications

Some people are allergic to lime flowers.

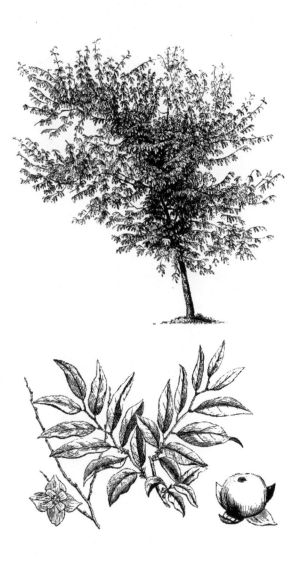

Lotus tree or Date plum *Diospyrus lotus*

According to Pant in 2010, people have used all parts of the *Diospyrus lotus* tree traditionally as medicine. According to Chopra in 1986 the seed is used as a sedative in traditional Chinese medicine, the fruit reduces fever and is used to promote secretions.

Mythology

Odysseus was blown off course as he was rounding Cape Malea at the southernmost tip of the Peloponnesus. On the tenth day they reached the land of the Lotus-eaters and landed to take in fresh water. He sent some of his men to see who lived on the island. When they did not return, he went to see what had happened to them and found them lying under the lotus trees, eating the lotus fruits and saying that they never wanted to go home. They just wanted to stay with the Lotus-eaters, eating the delicious fruit forever. Odysseus dragged them, protesting loudly, back to his ship, tied them under the ship's benches and set off. Interestingly in Greece the lotus fruit has a reputation for causing people to become forgetful if they eat too much of it. According to Ovid the lotus tree was sacred to the god Priapos, who pursued the Dryopian Nymph Lotis. She transformed herself into a lotus-tree to escape him.

Botanical Description

Diosperus lotus is a small, spreading, deciduous tree with glossy, dark green leaves up to 10 cm long. It grows up to 9 x 6 metres. Tiny, bell-shaped, greenish flowers appear in mid to late summer. The female flowers go on to produce yellow, plum-like fruit about 2 cm diameter, which turn purple when they are fully ripe. The fruit is delicious when perfectly ripe but is harsh and astringent before then. When dried the fruit tastes like dates.

Healing Properties

The leaves are used for lumbago, the fruits are carminative, astringent and cure biliousness, the seeds are sedative and the bark is bitter, astringent and reduces fever. Date plum leaves are antioxidant, analgesic, anti-inflammatory and protect the liver.

Chemical constituents

Diospyrus species contain many active compounds, including naphthoquinone, naphthalene and naphthol derivatives which are anti-bacterial, anti-fungal and anti-allergic, according to Waterman in 1979. In 1998 Ray found that diospyrin, a bisnaphthoquinone inhibited *Leishmania donovani*, a parasite which causes severe disease in humans living in the tropics. As far back as 1932, Watt isolated triterpenoids belonging to lupane, oleanane and ursane series from *Diospyrus lotus* and demonstrated that they were anti-inflammatory. *Diospyrus species* also contain lupeol, betulin and betulinic acid as well as β-sitosterol according to Herath in 1978. *Diospyrus lotus* fruits contain fatty acids and sugars, in addition to phenols, tannins, saponins and alkaloids.

Research

Phenolic compounds are an important natural source of anti-retrovirals for AIDS therapy because they are active against HIV-1 and are relatively non-toxic. In 2012 Rashed and team tested 7 phenolic compounds from *Diospyros lotus* fruits against HIV-1 and found that gallic acid was most active. In 2014 Gao found that extracts of phenolic compounds from Diospyros lotus fruits were antioxidant and free radical scavenging. Gallic acid was the most abundant phenolic compound and myricetin was the dominant flavonoid.

In 2015 Rauf isolated 3 new naphthaquinones from the roots of *Diospyrus lotus*. He demonstrated that these compounds prevented cancer cells from growing and spreading and were active against multi drug resistant cancer cells. Also, in 2015 he demonstrated the sedative and muscle relaxant effect of *Diospyrus lotus* roots *in vivo*. In 2017 Rauf demonstrated the sedative-hypnotic effect of a rare dimeric napthoquione from *Diospyrus lotus* roots. According to Gul in 2014, triterpenoids in this fruit are antioxidant, anti-allergic and anti-cancer and tannins in the fruit are more efficient than vitamin E. He found that tannins reduced high blood pressure and strokes in experimental animals. According to Chopra in 1992 Diospyrus lotus is sedative, astringent, laxative, nutritive, febrifuge, antitussive, antiseptic, anti-diabetic and anti-tumour.

I have been unable to find any clinical trials using *Diosperus lotus*, but people have been eating the fruits and using them as traditional medicine, as well as the leaves, bark and roots for a long time. I cannot recommend using the leaves, bark or roots, since there is no evidence that they are safe, but if you can find the fruits, eating them will undoubtedly be beneficial, not to mention delicious.

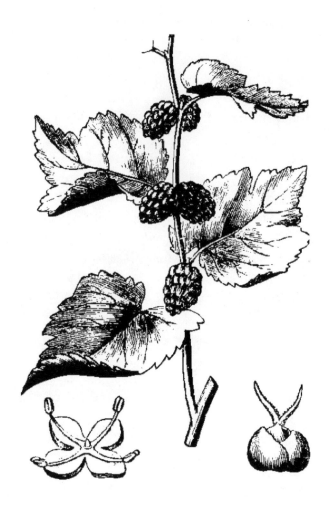

Mulberry black *Morus nigra*

When I lived in Italy, my husband and I bought an old olive mill, an enormous and somewhat derelict building which, like many old buildings in the Tuscan countryside, had seen several incarnations, one of which was as a silkworm producing enterprise. All that was left were two giant mulberry trees, whose leaves once fed thousands of silkworms and whose fruit, too high up to pick, used to drop onto the ground, leaving purple stains.

In Chinese markets, mulberry is often sold as a paste called as Sangshengao. People mix the paste into hot water to make tea to stimulate the liver and kidneys, to sharpen hearing and brighten eyes, according to Masilamani in 2008. People have used mulberry leaves traditionally to treat gastro-intestinal symptoms, hypertension, anaemia, kidney disease, liver and heart disease. They use the bark and roots to destroy internal parasites. People use the sap from the mulberry tree, which has a drying effect, to prevent tumours of the oral cavity from spreading, and for healing difficult wounds. Traditionally people brew mulberry leaf and chrysanthemum flower herbal tea to relieve the symptoms of fever, sore throat and dry eyes. They use the fruit syrup as a diaphoretic. Many people believe that a glass of mulberry wine daily helps to rid the blood of impurities.

Mythology

Ovid tells the tale of Pyramos and Thisbe, a pair of ill-fated lovers from the Assyrian city of Babylon. Their parents forbade their romance and the pair agreed to meet secretly beneath a white-berried mulberry tree outside the city limits. When Pyramos arrived, he found Thisbe's shawl in the jaws of a lion and believing her killed plunged a sword through his breast.

When Thisbe arrived and saw her dead lover, she killed herself. The mulberry tree soaked up the lovers' blood and its berries were turned from white to black-red. The Hamadryad Morea was the nymph of the mulberry-tree, according to Athenaeus.

Botanical Description

The black mulberry can grow up to 24 m high, forms a dense head of spreading branches, usually wider than the height of the tree. It has a short, rough trunk. The flowers are unisexual, the sexes in separate spikes, and grow as small, cylindrical, green separate catkins. The leaves grow alternately, are about 8 cm long, coarse, heart shaped with toothed edges, and can be hairy on top and downy underneath. The dark purple, oblong, 2.5 cm fruits look somewhat like blackberries, have short stalks and grow in fruit-clusters composed of little, closely packed drupes, each containing one seed and enclosed by 4 enlarged sepals, which have become succulent, thus forming the spurious berry.

Healing Properties

Mulberry fruit nourishes the skin and blood, benefits the liver and kidneys. The fresh fruits are a mild laxative and the fruit juice enhances health, calm the nerves, speeds up the metabolism of alcohol, balances internal secretions, enhances immunity and improves the cardiovascular system. Mulberry is an expectorant for bronchiectasis, chronic bronchitis and bronchial asthma.

Chemical constituents

Mulberries contain vitamins C, K1 and E, iron, potassium, high levels of phosphorus and many active compounds such as flavonoids, polyphenols, alkaloids, terpenoids, steroids, according to Scrivastava in 2003, Andallu in 2003 and Asano in 2001.

The fruits are a potent source of antioxidant anthocyanins. Cyanidin 3-rutinoside and cyanidin 3-glucoside are 2 anthocyanins in mulberry with strong anticancer properties.

Flavonoids and phenolic compounds in mulberry fruits include: apigenin, luteolin, quercetin, morin, caffeic acid, gallic acid, rutin, umbelliferone, chlorogenic acid and kaempferol.

The root bark contains an alkaloid, Deoxyjirimycin (DNJ), calcium malate, tannins, phytobaphenes, sugars, phytosterol, ceryl alcohol, fatty acids and phosphoric acid. Phenolic compounds in the twigs and root bark include maclurin, rutin, isoquercitrin, resveratrol and morin, according to Chang in 2011. The leaves contain flavonoids, anthocyanins, artocarpin, cycloartocarpin and analogues.

Research

Scientists all over the world have been studying mulberry and isolating active compounds from it. In 2008 Liu demonstrated that mulberries and mulberry extracts can reduce excess fat and lower cholesterol in animal studies. In 2011 Ting-Tsz found that mulberry fruits inhibited the accumulation of fats in some test tube experiments which, he suggested, might mean that the fruits could reduce the formation of fat in the liver, potentially helping prevent fatty liver disease.

In 2013 Chang demonstrated *in vitro* that anthocyanins in mulberries helped block fat formation, prevented fat accumulation and also promoted the clearance of fat out of the liver.

There has been a considerable amount of research into the potential healing properties of mulberry leaves, bark and roots, which have antioxidant, anti-diabetic, anti-AIDS properties as well as lowering blood pressure and preventing atherosclerosis. But all parts of the mulberry tree, apart from the fruit, are toxic, so although they are used traditionally in India, I have decided not to cover this research since it is not advisable to use these parts of the tree medicinally. I have however left the references to the research in the reference section, in case anyone is interested.

How to use Mulberry fruits

If you can find fresh mulberries they are packed with beneficial properties, but if you cannot find them you may be able to obtain dried mulberries which are also beneficial.

Contraindication

Diabetics should not eat mulberry fruits.

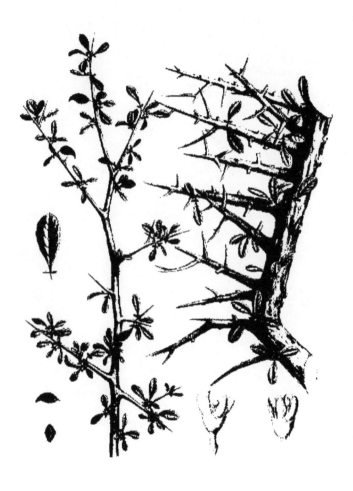

Myrrh tree *Commiphora myrrha*

Mythology

The myrrh tree is sacred to Aphrodite. Her followers used festal myrrh incense. According to Apollodorus, Antoninus Liberalis, and many others, the mother of Myrrha, the beautiful daughter of the King of Cyprus, dared to compare her beauty to the goddess Aphrodite. The goddess was highly offended and caused the girl to fall in love with her own father as punishment. When the King discovered that his daughter had seduced him in disguise, he chased after her, with an axe, screaming murderous threats, but the goddess mercifully intervened and transformed Myrrha into a myrrh tree. Myrrha was pregnant when she became a tree and gave birth to Adonis from her trunk. The Nymphs took the new born baby and brought him up. Myrrha's tears oozed from the trunk of the tree to form the aromatic gum, myrrh.

According to Herodotus:

> *"Arabia is the only country which produces frankincense, myrrh, cassia, and cinnamon..., the trees bearing the frankincense are guarded by winged serpents of small size and various colours."*

Diodorus Siculus wrote, in the second half of the 1st century BCE, that:

> *"All of Arabia exudes a most delicate fragrance; even the seamen passing by Arabia can smell the strong fragrance that gives health and vigour."*

There are 54 references to myrrh as incense and many references to it as a component in the mixtures used to treat wounds, sepsis and worms in the Hippocratic corpus. This may have been because it was used to treat battle wounds, for as we know, the

Greeks were constantly fighting battles. Dioscorides prescribed myrrh or its oils for infections of the mouth, teeth and eyes. It was recommended for cough, particularly cough in children. This was one of the earliest specific paediatric prescriptions.

There is a long history of trade in myrrh and frankincense, which were both considered as valuable as gold, as evidenced by the three Magi who brought gifts of gold, frankincense and myrrh to the infant Jesus. These precious substances were transported over land and sea from the desert regions where they were painstakingly collected by local tribes. As long ago as 3,000 BCE myrrh was probably being traded in Egypt and beyond, transported by donkeys to Jerusalem and Egypt from the Dhofar region of what is today Oman, through Yemen, turning north to follow the Red Sea coast. When people began to domesticate the camel in about 1100 BCE the 'Incense Trade' grew, as camels could transport greater loads across the desert lands of the Arabian peninsula.

Botanical Description

Myrrh is a small, spiny desert tree not more than 3 m high, native to Arabia and the horn of Africa. Its knotted branches and branchlets stick out at right-angles, ending in a sharp spine. It has scanty, small, unequal, oval, trifoliate leaves. There are ducts in the bark and the tissue between them breaks down, forming large cavities which fill up with a granular secretion. People make cuts in the bark to release it and it flows out as a pale-yellow liquid which hardens to a reddish-brown mass. The pieces are brittle, with a granular structure, semi-transparent and oily. It has a characteristically bitter taste: '*murr*' is Arabic for bitter.

Healing Properties

Myrrh is pungent, astringent, aromatic, strongly stimulant, antiseptic, expectorant and anti-spasmodic. It also stimulates the uterus. The European Medicines Agency say that myrrh can be used to treat minor ulcers and inflammation in the mouth and minor wounds and small boils. It is often added to oral preparations and people use it as a mouth wash, according to Wallis in 1967 and Trease and Evans in 1989. It is one of the most effective herbal medicines for treating sore throats, mouth ulcers, gingivitis and extreme ulceration. Tincture of myrrh is used to treat aphthous ulcers (blisters inside the mouth) according to Pesko in 1990. British herbalist, Chevallier recommends using the tincture (diluted in water) to treat inflammation of the bone, connective tissue, and gum surrounding and supporting the teeth, usually caused by bacteria that grow in the spaces between the gum and lower part of the tooth crown. He also advises his patients to use it to treat catarrh, pharyngitis and sinusitis, chronic gastritis, laryngitis and respiratory complaints. Herbalists Bown and Chevallier use it to relieve spasms, inflammation and digestive discomfort and to encourage healing. People take the resin internally to treat dyspepsia and bronchial infections, glandular fever, tonsillitis, pharyngitis, gingivitis, menstrual and circulatory problems. Myrrh is antiseptic for wounds and abrasions. The mild astringency makes it a useful treatment for acne, boils and mild inflammatory skin problems, according to Vander Zanden in 1980. People use it to treat chronic bronchitis and bronchial asthma. It is used in traditional Chinese medicine to relieve pain and swelling due to traumatic injury, according to Lee in 1993. It can be used to lower cholesterol in the blood according to Jain in 1994.

Chemical constituents

Myrrh contains a 2-8% volatile oil, 23-40% resin and 40-60% gum. The volatile oil contains cadinene, elemol, eugenol, cuminaldehyde, numerous furano-sesquiterpenes, as well as furanoeudesma-1,3-diene and many other compounds. Myrrh resin contains alpha-, beta- and gamma-commiphoric acid, esters of a resin acid, and 2 phenolic resins, alpha- and beta-heerabomyrrhol and alpha and beta-heerabomyrrholic acids and many other compounds.

The gum contains proteoglycans, diterpenes sesquiterpenes, lactones, including commiferin and steroids among other compounds.

Research

There has been a great deal of research over the years into the healing properties of Myrrh, most of it carried out in the laboratory. I'm only going to mention a small part of it, for although these experiments demonstrate that various components of myrrh have many different healing properties, until someone carries out large scale clinical trials, we will not have scientific evidence that it works in human subjects. Of course, herbalists have been using it for many centuries and observing the results in their patients.

In 1987 Al Awadi and Gumaa found that Myrrh gum extract prevented high blood sugar in both normal and diabetic rats. They suggested in 1991 that it might be useful for treating non-insulin dependent diabetes. Several researchers, including Arora in 1973, Lata in 1991 and Michie in 1991, demonstrated that myrrh extracts decreased cholesterol, phospholipids, triglycerides and lipids in the blood of various experimental high cholesterol animals. In 1999 Olajide found that myrrh extract protected mice from thrombosis.

In 1998 Atta found that myrrh extract was anti-inflammatory and lowered the temperature of mice. Several scientists, including Quereshi in 1993 Al Harbi in 1994, demonstrated the anti-tumour effect of myrrh *in vivo*. In 1997 Al Harbi demonstrated that myrrh protected mice from damage caused by indomethacin.

The terpenoids (especially furano-sesquiterpenes), in myrrh essential oil, are antiseptic, anaesthetic and anti-tumour. In

2000 Dolara demonstrated that the sesquiterpene fractions were anti-bacterial, anti-fungal and local anaesthetic. In 1978 Sarbhoy demonstrated that the essential oil of myrrh was anti-fungal. In 1977 Narain Sharma demonstrated that myrrh was anti-inflammatory *in vivo*. In 1984 Tripathi demonstrated that myrrh stimulated the thyroid gland in rats. Hasan in 1989 stated that myrrh can be used to regulate menses. In 1988 Kubec patented a cosmetic preparation for treating hair and scalp.

In 2011 El-Sherbiny and El-Sherbiny carried out a small clinical trial, treating women suffering from metronidazole-resistant Trichomoniasis, a common venereal disease, with myrrh or with pomegranate extracts. Both herbal treatments were effective in 80% of cases. In 2009 Rashad reviewed the clinical trials which gave myrrh to patients suffering with schistosomiasis, a parasitic disease which is very common in Egypt. He found that myrrh effectively kills the parasite and it also kills the snails which the parasite lives in, its secondary host. Unfortunately, there will never be enough myrrh to treat all the people suffering from schistosomiasis in Egypt.

Behcet's disease is rare. Symptoms include genital and mouth ulcers, red, painful eyes and blurred vision, acne-like spots, headaches and painful, stiff and swollen joints. In 2017 Albishri carried out a small study at Tadawi clinic in Taif, in Saudi Arabia. He gave 16 patients with Behcet's disease a myrrh mouthwash 4 times a day for a week. 50 percent of the patients reported complete pain relief and 18.75 percent said that their ulcers disappeared. This was a very small study, looking at treatment for only one symptom of a rare disease.

Probably the most interesting research so far into the healing properties of myrrh was carried out in China, where in 2020 Bailly reviewed a traditional Chinese medicine, Xihuang pills (XHP). XHP contains frankincense, myrrh, musk (*Moschus moschiferus*) and bezoar (*Calculus bovis*) and is used to treat cancer. The Chinese use XHP to limit the spread of the cancer and to protect non-tumour cells from damage caused by conventional treatments. According to traditional Chinese medicine, frankincense and myrrh promote blood and vital energy circulation and decrease swelling and pain, musk activates stagnant blood and vital energy circulation and bezoar detoxifies. The Chinese have been using XHP to treat cancer for a long time.

Several scientists tested XHP in the laboratory and found that it stopped breast cancer cells from growing and spreading. In 2019 Mao analysed 13 clinical trials which included 1,272 patients who were treated with XHP alone or in combination with chemotherapy (636 each). He concluded that XHP reduced the adverse effects of chemotherapy, especially nausea and vomiting. He also noted that the patients' immune systems were stimulated: CD3 and CD4 immune cells increased in the patients treated with XHP and chemotherapy.

How to Use Myrrh

Many myrrh preparations are available: tincture, powder, essential oil, as well as gum and resin. As you can see from the chemistry, the different preparations contain different compounds and therefore have different properties. Herbalists tend to use a high alcohol tincture, but this has to be stored under special conditions to prevent it from bursting into flames. The tincture contains resins and is strongly anti-bacterial. Diluted in water it makes a good mouth wash. Alternatively, you can make a mouthwash by adding 500 mg - 1.25 g of gum resin to boiling water and leaving to steep for 15 minutes. Strain and use to treat gingivitis and mouth ulcers, or gargle with it to relieve sore throat, to alleviate bronchial catarrh, coughs and colds.

Use a ground up powder of myrrh to dust on wounds, haemorrhoids, oozing skin conditions and bed sores, to speed up the healing process. Take capsules containing 400-500 mg of ground myrrh 2-3 times a day to treat dyspepsia and bronchial infections, tonsillitis, pharyngitis, menstrual and circulatory problems. Mix a few drops of myrrh essential oil with a carrier oil such as almond and use to massage painful joints. Make a vapour rub with 4 drops of myrrh essential oil and a tablespoon of coconut oil. Rub onto your chest to relieve coughs, colds and congestion.

Contraindications

Don't use myrrh during pregnancy because it may cause a miscarriage. Always dilute myrrh before use. Some people are allergic to myrrh.

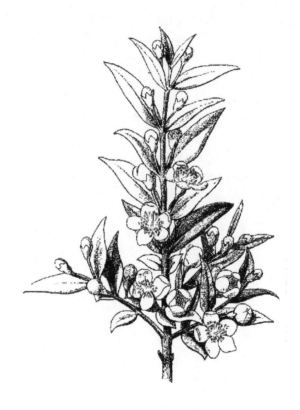

Myrtle *Myrtus communis*

The Unani System of Medicine has been using common myrtle since the time of the ancient Greeks. Unani healers use the berries, leaves and essential oil for gastric ulcer, diarrhoea, dysentery, vomiting, rheumatism, haemorrhages, sinusitis and leucorrhoea (a whitish or yellowish discharge of mucus from the vagina.)

Mythology

Myrtle was sacred to Aphrodite, goddess of love, beauty and sex, who is often depicted with a myrtle crown, sprig or wreath. Myrtle trees were planted in her temple gardens and shrines. Brides wore myrtle-garlands and bathed in myrtle-scented water on their wedding day. Aphrodite's myrtle nymphs raised the baby Aeacus, god of beekeeping, olive curing and cheesemaking. Bees flock to the myrtle tree, which blooms late and provides surplus honey for the bees' dormant period. Myrtle honey was once used medicinally.

According to Stuart in 1994, Hippocrates, Pliny and Dioscorides all sing the praises of myrtle. Dioscorides described how to prepare myrtle oil and prescribed an extract in wine for lung and bladder infections.

Botanical Description

Myrtle has an upright stem, 2.4 3 m high, its branches form a close full head, thickly covered with evergreen leaves. Its stem is branched and the dark green leaves are thick, stiff, glossy, smooth, hairless, ovate to lanceolate and grow opposite each other in pairs, or whorled. They are aromatic, with smooth edges and 2.5-3.8 cm long, without glands on the blade of the leaf. Myrtle has stiff white flowers about 2 cm diameter that grow from an axil on slender stalks, with yellow anthers. The petals are pure white with glands and somewhat hairy edges. They give off a sweet fragrant smell. The berries are 0.7-1.2 cm, about the size of a pea, round or ovoid-ellipsoid, blue-black or white with hard kidney shaped seeds. They start off pale green, then turn deep red and finally become dark indigo when fully mature. They are bitter when unripe, sweet when ripe.

Healing Properties

The leaves are astringent, antiseptic, laxative, and lower blood sugar, according to Trease and Evans in 2006; analgesic according to Kirtikar in 1988. They are aromatic, balsamic, tonic and stop blood flow from wounds. The root is anti-bacterial according to Agarwal in 1986. People use myrtle to treat urinary infections, digestive problems, bronchial congestion, and dry coughs. They use it externally to treat wounds, gum infections and haemorrhoids. Essential oil of myrtle leaves is antiseptic and is used to treat acne and rheumatism.

The fruit is antiseptic, carminative, astringent and emmenagogue, according to Nadkarni in 1989; and used to treat dysentery, diarrhoea, haemorrhoids and ulcers. It is soothing and analgesic, and stops the flow of blood from wounds, according to Baitar in 1999. In 1920 Ghani stated that the berries were a tonic for the heart, stomach and brain and were diuretic and would break up kidney stones and stop vomiting. They are anti-inflammatory and protect the kidneys, according to Hakeem in 1895.

Chemical constituents

The plant contains a wide range of biologically active compounds such as tannins, flavonoids, coumarins, fixed oil, sugars, citric acid, malic acid and antioxidants as well as high quantities of vitamins and essential oil. Almost all the volatile compounds in the essential oil are terpenes and terpene alcohols: 1,8-cineole, α-pinene, myrtenyl acetate, limonene, linalool and α-terpinolene. The essential oil is extracted from the leaves, branches, fruits and flowers through steam distillation, according to Nadkarni in 1989. The main active compounds in myrtle leaves are polyphenols, Myrtucommulone (MC) and semi-myrtucommulone (S-MC), unique compounds.

The major compounds in the berries are phenolic compounds, flavonoids and anthocyanins. They contain citric acid, malic acid, resin, tannin, fixed oil and 14 fatty acids, including oleic (67.07%) palmitic (10.24%) and stearic acid (8.19%), according to Serce in 2010.

The seeds contain 12-15% fatty oil consisting of glycerides of oleic, linoleic, myristic, palmitic, linolenic and lauric acid, according to Rastogi in 1991.

The roots contain tannins, alkaloids, glycosides, reducing sugars, fixed oil, gallic acids, phenolic acids, quercetin and patuletin, according to Diaz in 1987.

Research

Several scientists, including Alem in 2008 have demonstrated that myrtle extract is anti-bacterial and anti-fungal. In 1989 Al-Hindawi found that extracts of myrtle were anti-inflammatory *in vivo*. In 2005 Feisst demonstrated *in vitro* and *in vivo* that MC, S-MC are anti-inflammatory. In 2008 Rosa and team demonstrated that MC and S-MC from myrtle fruits protected low density lipoproteins and polyunsaturated fats and cholesterol from oxidative damage. They suggested that these compounds could protect humans from atherosclerosis. In 2010 Serce demonstrated that myrtle fruit extracts were antioxidant and free radical scavenging *in vitro*. Also, in 2010 Amensour found that extracts of both berries and leaves were antioxidant, the leaves more than the berries. Also, in 2010 Mimica-Dukic demonstrated that the essential oil of myrtle was free radical scavenging *in vitro*.

In 1984 Elfellah and team demonstrated that myrtle extract

reduced high blood sugar in mice. In 2004 Sepici found leaf extracts as well as essential oil from the myrtle leaf reduced blood sugar in rabbits. In 2007 Dineel demonstrated that myrtle oil reduced glucose absorption in rabbits. In 2009 Fahim demonstrated that phenolic compounds extracted from myrtle leaves were anti-diabetic in rats.

In 2010 Mimica-Dukic demonstrated *in vitro* that myrtle essential oil protected cells from mutating. In 2008 Hayder and team isolated myricetin-3-o-galactoside and myricetin-3-o-rhamnoside from myrtle leaves and demonstrated that these compounds protected cells from mutating and from oxidative stress and helped cells to repair DNA damage.

In 1985 Al-Zohyri and team demonstrated that myrtle leaf extract made the heart beat more slowly and more strongly *in vivo*. In 2009 Salouage demonstrated that myrtle extracts protected the livers of rats. In 2010 Sumbul and team demonstrated that extracts of myrtle dried berries protected rats from ulcers.

Repeated aphthous stomatitis (RAS) (the repeated formation of mouth ulcers), is common and painful. In 2010 Babaee carried out a randomized, double-blind, clinical trial with a novel paste containing myrtle, which is used traditionally in Iran to treat mouth ulcers. He treated half of the 45 patients with RAS with placebo paste and half with myrtle oral paste. Subjects applied the paste 4 times a day for 6 days. Patients who used the myrtle paste said that their ulcers improved, they felt less pain, less inflammation. There were no side effects.

In 2017 Slimeni and team gave extracts of myrtle fruit to half of 32 male and female athletes and placebo to the other half for 4 weeks. They measured lipid, protein, mineral levels in blood samples before and after exercise and found that those taking the myrtle extract increased their performance. They also found that proteins and iron increased significantly while triglycerides decreased. They concluded that the phenolic compounds in myrtle and the antioxidant properties of the fruit help to increase athletic performance and that possibly athletes could take myrtle fruit extracts to prevent muscle damage. However, it was a small trial, so larger trials would need to be carried out before actively promoting myrtle supplements for athletes.

In 2016 Masoudi carried out a randomised clinical trial on 120 married women aged 18-40 years who suffered from bacterial vaginosis. They were randomly divided into 3 groups of 40 participants. One group was given a vaginal gel containing metronidazole and extract of *Myrtus communis L* leaves, one group was given a vaginal gel containing metronidazole and *Berberis vulgaris* and a third group was just given a metronidazole vaginal gel. They applied the gel for 5 nights. The results showed that vaginal gel with extracts of *Myrtus communis* or *Berberis vulgaris* in metronidazole base were more effective than metronidazole alone on bacterial vaginosis without any serious side effect or relapse. 30% of patients using only metronidazole experienced relapse during 3 weeks follow up. Although this was a small trial the results are interesting, since they demonstrate that some plant extracts can be used together with pharmaceutical drugs to good effect.

In 2015 Zohalinezhad carried out a 6-week double-blind randomised clinical trial on patients who all suffered from gastro-oesophageal reflux disease (FSSG). He divided the 45 patients into 3 groups. He gave one group myrtle berry extract 1000 mg/d, a second group omeprazol capsules, 20 mg/d, and third group a combination of berry extract and omeprazol. All 3 groups improved. It would be a good idea to carry out further and larger studies.

Although the myrtle plant has so many active constituents and such promising therapeutic possibilities, there have been few clinical trials, apart from these 4 above. It would appear that scientists are more interested in isolating compounds with interesting activity which could be developed by the pharmaceutical industry.

How to use Myrtle

Use myrtle essential oil in a vaporiser to ease chronic bronchial and lung conditions, to help expel phlegm from the lungs and bronchi, to aid sleep. Use it to help people suffering from withdrawal from addiction to drugs and to soothe and ease self-destructive behaviour and feelings of anger, fear, greed and envy.

Mix with a carrier oil and use in aromatherapy to treat physical exhaustion, anxiety, insomnia, depression, nervous tension and stress.

Blend a few drops into a cream to correct over-dry or over oily skin and to eradicate acne. Make an ointment with witch hazel, cypress essential oil and myrtle essential oil for an astringent effect on piles.

Make a tea with myrtle leaves to treat bronchial congestion and dry cough. Use as a vaginal wash to treat bacterial and yeast infections.

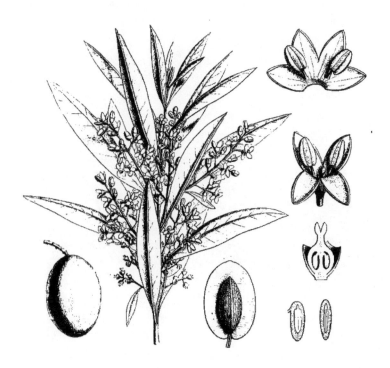

Olive tree *Olea europaea*

Years ago, when I lived in Italy, I had an olive grove on a steep, terraced hillside. Every year in November my sister and I went to pick the olives, spreading out nets under the trees and scrambling about on the icy branches combing the olives off so that they fell in a pattering rain onto the nets below. When we had picked the whole crop, we took the bags of olives to the press, an old-fashioned cold press where the olives were ground into a paste with water, then spread onto round mats which were stacked one above the other on a long metal pole, above which the press loomed. After pressing, the resultant dirty looking mixture was whirled round in a centrifuge to separate out the oil. People who brought their olives to be pressed came with slices of bread which they held under the tap from which the freshly pressed oil dripped, so that they could taste it, green, pungent and full of healing properties.

Mythology

The most sacred olive tree grew in Athene's sanctuary on the Acropolis of Athens. According to Apollodorus, Pausanias, Hyginus and Ovid, Athene and Poseidon once engaged in a contest for dominion of Athens. Zeus agreed to award the city to the god who produced the best gift for man. Athene created the first olive tree which sprang from the rock of the Acropolis, whilst Poseidon produced a horse. The gods judged Athene's the better gift and awarded her the city. Athene was fond of an Athenian girl, Moria. When she died the goddess transformed her into a sacred olive tree (*moria*).

The official seal and emblem of the World Health Organisation features the rod of Asclepius over a world map surrounded by olive tree branches, chosen as a symbol of peace and health.

Victors at the Olympian Games were crowned with wild olive.

Botanical Description

Olea europaea is a small, evergreen tree which can grow up to 20 m high, with pale grey bark, thin branches with opposite branchlets and shortly stalked, opposite, lanceolate, pointed, smooth leaves, pale green above and silvery below. It has numerous small, creamy white flowers. The fruit is an ovoid drupe. I think everyone knows what an olive looks like.

Healing Properties

In traditional medicine, olive leaves are used to fight colds, flu, yeast infections, viral infections, shingles and herpes. Olive leaves are used to support the heart, to treat high blood pressure, gout, arteriosclerosis and rheumatism. *Olea europaea* leaves bring down blood pressure and high temperature, stimulate the production of bile, are diuretic, laxative, skin cleanser, and also are used to treat urinary infections, gallstones, bronchial asthma and diarrhoea.

Chemical constituents

Olive leaves contain oleuropein, a secoiridoid glucoside with a multitude of useful properties. Two of its by-products are also present in the rest of the olive plant: demethyl-oleuropein and the oleoside methyl ester. These two compounds increase as the olives ripen, while the quantity of oleuropein decreases. The leaves also contain glycosides, flavonoids, poly-unsaturated fatty acids and the anti-viral calcium elenolate. Olives also contain ligstroside, oleuroside, cornoside and esters of tyrosol and hydroxyl-tyrosol.

Research

Many scientists have carried out research to prove that olive is antioxidant, anti-viral, anti-microbial, anti-diabetic and has potential for use for cardiovascular disorders.

As far back as 1854 Daniel Hanbury wrote that he had used a

tincture of olive leaf successfully to treat severe cases of fever and malaria. In the early 19th century Spanish physicians sometimes prescribed olive leaves to bring down fever and consequently during the Spanish war of 1808-1813 the French Officers de Sante often used olive leaf tincture to treat cases of 'intermittent fever' (malaria). The British soon discovered this method and used it to treat sick Britons returning from tropical colonies.

Decades later, scientists isolated a bitter substance from the leaf, which they believed helped the olive tree to resist insects and bacteria, and called it oleuropein. It is in olive oil and in every part of the tree and is the bitter material that is eliminated from olives when they are cured. In 2005 De Nino determined the quantity of oleuropein in olive oil. Oil from Calabria, Italy contains significant amounts of oleuropein, ranging from 1 ppm to 11 ppm.

In 1972 Petkov demonstrated that oleuropein was anti-bacterial. In 1999 Bisignano discovered that it stimulated macrophages (important cells of the immune system that engulf and destroy bacteria.) In 1995 Chimi demonstrated that olive leaf extract and oleuropein and caffeic acid were antioxidant. In 1994 Visioli reported that oleuropein prevented the oxidation of LDL cholesterol. Oxidised LDL is the most damaging form of cholesterol and can start the damage to the blood vessels, leading to atherosclerosis. In 1992 Gonzales found that olive leaf extracts lowered cholesterol *in vivo*. In 1994 Visoli demonstrated that oleuropein prevented fats from accumulating in the bloodstream of a mouse, and suggested that it may help to prevent cardiovascular diseases by preventing atherosclerotic plaques from forming in blood vessels. In 1995 Petroni demonstrated that olive leaf inhibited the clumping together of platelets, which can lead to clots forming. Several scientists, including Zaslaver in 2005, Benavente-Garcia in 2000, Briante in 2002, demonstrated that olive leaf extracts were antioxidant *in vitro* and *in vivo*. In 2006 Al-Azzawie found that oleuropein was antioxidant in rabbits. In 1999 Bennani-Kabchi demonstrated that olive leaf extract lowered blood sugar in rats. The active constituent was oleuropein. Both Gonzalez in 1992 and Al-Azzawie in 2006 demonstrated that oleuropein lowered blood sugar *in vivo*.

In 1991 Zarzuelo demonstrated that an olive leaf extract dilated blood vessels in a laboratory study. Oleuropeoside was the compound responsible for the relaxant effect. He also found that oleuropein lowered blood pressure and olive extracts were anti-spasmodic, vasodilator, and anti-arrhythmic in the laboratory. In 1996 Pieroni demonstrated that olive leaf was anti-inflammatory *in vitro*.

In 1999 Bisignano found that hydroxy-tyrosol had broad spectrum anti-microbial activity, as potent as ampicillin and erythromycin. Several scientists have demonstrated that olive leaf extract is anti-viral, including Soret in 1969, Renis in 1970 and Heinze in 1975, who all reported that calcium elenolate, was the compound responsible for the anti-viral effect. Calcium elenolate inhibits several viruses *in vitro*, including rhinovirus, which causes the common cold, myxoviruses, Herpes viruses, encephalo-myocarditis, polio viruses, two strains of leukemia virus, many strains of influenza and para-influenza viruses, according to Renis in 1975.

The renin-angiotensin system controls blood pressure. Angiotensin converting enzyme converts angiotensin I to angiotensin II, which stimulates the blood vessels to constrict which raises blood pressure. In 1996 Hansen reported that olive leaf extract inhibited both angiotensin converting enzymes.

In 2002 Al-Qarawi demonstrated that olive leaf extract stimulated the thyroid gland in rats.

Clinical trials

Clinical studies have consistently demonstrated that the people who live on a Mediterranean diet, rich in olive oil, fruits, vegetables and grains, have a lower-than-average risk of coronary heart disease, according to Kushi in 1995.

In 1949 Capretti and Bonaconza gave human adult patients 5 ml of an olive leaf infusion or 3 ml of an olive leaf decoction to drink once daily for 20-25 days. They noticed a diuretic effect.

High blood pressure is a harmful disease that develops unnoticed over time. Ideally it should be diagnosed early and the patient should make lifestyle changes rather than taking harmful drugs. In 2008 Perrinjaquet-Moccetti and team carried out an open study on 40 monozygotic twins with borderline high blood pressure. They gave 500 or 1000 mg/day of olive leaf extract (EFLA R 943), to each pair of twins in one group for 8 weeks or advice on a favourable lifestyle to another group of twins. Blood pressure decreased significantly within pairs, depending on the dose of olive leaf extract.

In 2011 Susalit carried out a double-blind, randomised, parallel and active-controlled clinical study to find out whether an olive leaf extract (EFLA R 943) would lower blood pressure, in patients with stage 1 high blood pressure. They gave half the patients 500 mg of olive leaf extract orally twice daily for 8 weeks. They gave the control 12.5 mg Captopril twice daily. After 8 weeks of treatment, blood pressure of both groups fell. Triglycerides levels also fell in the group who took the olive leaf extract but not in the Captopril group. The olive leaf extract contained 18-26% (m/m) oleuropein, 30-40% (m/m) polyphenols as well as verbascoside and luteolin-7-glucoside.

In 2012 Weinstein and team carried out a controlled clinical trial with 79 adults with type 2 diabetes. They gave half the patients a 500 mg olive leaf extract tablet per day and placebo to the other half for 14 weeks. The blood sugar and insulin of the subjects treated with olive leaf extract fell.

In 2013 de Bock and team carried out a randomised, double-blinded, placebo-controlled, crossover trial with 46 overweight men. He gave half the patients olive leaf extract capsules containing 51.1 mg oleuropein and 9.7 mg hydroxytyrosol per day, and the other half a placebo for 12 weeks. They found that the group who took the olive leaf had significantly improved insulin sensitivity, suggesting that olive leaf extract may help to prevent type 2 diabetes.

Conclusions

Olive oil is good for you. But make sure that you obtain cold pressed organic olive oil for the maximum health benefit. In Mediterranean countries people drizzle olive oil onto salads, soups, cooked vegetables, rice, pasta and many other dishes, relishing the taste of it. Olive leaf extract has many healing properties and has been used traditionally as medicine for many years. The European Medicine Authority say that since people have been using olive leaf for a long time, they can allow its use to promote water elimination through the kidneys. They do not recommend it for anything else. But herbalists use olive leaf to treat many other conditions.

How to use olive leaf

Take olive leaf to normalise blood pressure. If your blood pressure is abnormally high you should consult a doctor but if it is only slightly raised you could take olive leaf to lower it. You could take olive leaf to stimulate your immune system.

Dosage

Liquid olive leaf extract: 30 - 50 drops, 3 times daily
98 ml liquid contains 182g extract, 1 g = 28 drops
Coated tablet for oral use: 3-5 coated tablets containing 14 mg dry extract each divided into 2-3 single doses.
Hard capsules (containing 275 mg powder each) 3 - 5 times daily.

Contraindications

People with low blood pressure or taking blood pressure lowering medications should not take olive leaf extract. Anyone with hypoglycaemia or taking insulin should not take olive leaf extract. Olive leaf may conflict with some antibiotics.

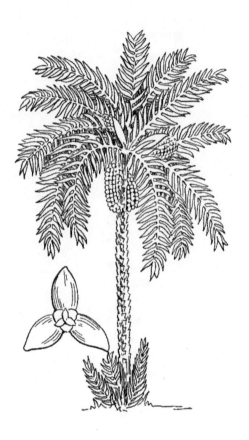

Palm date *Phoenix dactylifera*

Traditionally people use dates to treat fever, anaemia, asthma, bronchitis, cancer, catarrh, cough, diarrhoea, fatigue, fever, flu, gonorrhoea, piles, sterility, stomach ache, toothache, vaginitis, warts and whitlow according to Duke and Wain in 1981.

Mythology

According to the Homeric Hymns, the goddess Hera, Zeus's jealous wife, relentlessly pursued the goddess Leto, who was either Zeus's former wife, his concubine or merely one of his victims, since he ravaged every beautiful female he laid eyes on. Pregnant with the twins Apollo and Artemis, Leto eventually landed on the floating island of Delos, where she gave birth to Apollo whilst clinging to a date palm beside the Inopos River. As soon as Leto touched down on the island, it became fixed and when Apollo grew up, he had a sacred palm tree in his sanctuary there. Nike, the goddess of victory, held a palm branch as an attribute.

Description

A medium sized tree which grows to a height of 15-25 m. Compound leaves are 4-8 m long, with pointed leaflets arranged on either side of the stem, in pairs opposite each other, folded or rolled inward, with a terminal crown of 100-120 leaves. It has small, white flowers on richly branched spikes arranged round a fleshy axis, surrounded by a solitary large sheathing bract. The flowers have a cup-shaped calyx with toothed petals, in female flowers twice as long as the calyx. They have 6 stamens and 3 ovaries, only one of which develops into fruit. The fruits are 2.5-7.5 cm long, with fleshy, sugary pericarp, yellowish to reddish brown.

Healing Properties

Dates are high in fibre so they help to maintain a healthy digestive system. They provide the body with much needed minerals and vitamins. They are high in antioxidants which protect the body's cells from damage which can lead to ill health, including heart disease, Alzheimers and cancer. Since they contain high levels of anti-inflammatory compounds, they may protect the brain from neuro-degeneration and the development of plaques which cause Alzheimers. Eating dates during the last few weeks of pregnancy may promote cervical dilation and lower the need for induced labor. They may also be helpful for reducing labour time and prevent post-delivery bleeding because they contain some constricting substances. Since dates contain phosphorus, potassium, calcium and magnesium, all minerals required for healthy bones, they may help to prevent osteoporosis. Dates may prevent the formation of kidney stones due to their diuretic and anti-inflammatory actions and since they contain vitamins E and C and melatonin, they may help protect the kidneys. Dates contain plenty of potassium, so they can help alleviate potassium deficiency, a common problem often caused by diuretics. Although dates are very sweet their high fibre content results in a low glycemic index because the sugars in them are released into the blood stream slowly.

Chemical constituents

Dates contain protein, carbohydrate, fibre, a rich array of minerals: potassium, calcium, phosphorus, iron, zinc, boron, cobalt, copper, fluorine, magnesium, manganese, phosphorous and sodium. In many varieties, there may be as much as 0.9% potassium in the flesh and 0.5% in some seeds. Dates also contain selenium, another element believed to help prevent cancer and important in immune function. They contain the vitamins: beta carotene, thiamine, riboflavin, niacin and vitamin C, as well as tannins, saponins, cardiac glycoside and steroids. The protein in dates contains 23 types of amino acids, including glycine and threonine. Dates contain a huge number of different poly-phenolic compounds, which protect the body from ill-health, including cancer. The plant produces these compounds as defence against UV light and pathogens. Dates contain 19 different flavonoid glycosides of luteolin, quercetin, and apigenin in methylated and sulfated forms, making dates the only fruit or vegetable known to contain flavonoid sulfates. The pollen contains cholesterol and estrone. The sorocarp contains cholesterol, ampesterol, stigmasterol, beta-sitosterol and isofucosterol. The seed contains fatty acids.

Research

In recent years, an explosion of interest in the health benefits of dates has led to many *in vitro* and animal studies and the identification of chemical compounds in dates. I am not going to cover all the research that was carried out in laboratories, but just mention a few studies. Scientists hypothesise that the vast array of polyphenolic compounds in dates have formed due to exposure to extreme temperatures. They theorise that we benefit from the synergy among these polyphenolic compounds, which far outweigh the benefits of any singular polyphenol. And The World Health Organisation has stated that there is evidence to suggest that consuming plenty of polyphenols may decrease the risk of developing cancer but, hedging their bets, they say that there is insufficient evidence to prove this.

In 2005 Al Farsi demonstrated that dates contain antioxidant and anti-mutagenic properties. Isruda and John in 2005 observed that extracts of polysaccharides from dates prevented Sarcoma tumour cells from growing in mice. In 2002 Vayalil reported that date extracts were anti-mutagenic and antioxidant. In 2005 Allaith demonstrated that date extracts inhibited the oxidation of fats and proteins and were potent free radical scavengers. In 2009 Panahi and Asadi reported that date extract controlled blood cholesterol levels and protected nerves from oxidative injury *in vivo*. In 2004 Mohammed and Al-Okbi showed that date extracts were anti-inflammatory and suppressed swelling in the foot and arthritis *in vivo*. Several scientists, including Al-Qarawi in 2004 and Mohammed in 2008 found that date extracts protected rats from liver damage. Date extract counteracts the effect of alcohol intoxication, according to Thornfeldt in 2006. In 2009 Ayachi reported that dates were anti-bacterial.

In 2003 Al Qarawi demonstrated that date extracts stimulated food to transit through rats faster. On the other hand, in 2008, Al-Taher demonstrated that date extracts had an antidiarrheal effect in rats. In 2005 Al-Qarawi demonstrated that dates protected rats from ulcers. In 1995 Elgasim found that date extracts increased the sperm count in guinea pigs and stimulated an increase in testosterone in rats.

In 2019 Nasiri reviewed the clinical trials that had been carried out to examine the effects of eating dates during pregnancy. They found that date consumption significantly reduced gestation duration, increased dilation of the cervix when women were admitted to hospital and shortened the first stage of labour.

Conclusions

Dates are a wonderful food, packed with beneficial compounds. They may help to prevent cancer, heart disease and many other forms of ill health but the lack of clinical trials means that there is insufficient evidence for any of these health benefits. People living in countries where dates grow eat vast quantities of them without any apparent ill effects. As long as we continue to import them, we can continue to enjoy these delicious fruits.

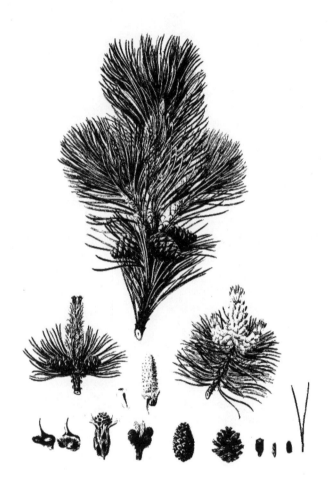

Pine Aleppo and Pine Turkish *Pinus halepensis* and *Pinus brutia*

In 2004 Lentini mentioned that several plant exudates, including pine resins, were discovered during archeological excavations at Pyrgos–Mavrorachi, a 19th century BCE Bronze age site near the south-coast of Cyprus. So clearly the ancient Greeks were using pine resins and they were using them as medicine, as evidenced by Dioscorides' De Materia Medica, which mentions several pine resins. According to Berendes in 1902 Dioscorides says that one of the properties common to all resins was their warming effect, in particular "burnt" resin in plasters or ointments to treat rheumatic conditions. A plaster was made from pounded pine resin dissolved in hot barley gruel, which was then spread on a piece of cloth the size of the affected area, such as the knee, ankle, or hand. This would increase blood flow to the area where it was applied, thus effectively 'warming' the area. The plaster might also have analgesic and anti-inflammatory effects.

Paulus Aegineta mentioned turpentine poultices for treating rheumatic diseases and gout, according to Adams in 1844. In 1985 Arnold-Apostolides recorded several medicinal uses for resin and tar from *P. brutia* and *P. halepensis,* applied topically. In 1996 Honda reported that people in western Anatolia also used the resin from *P. nigra* and *P. brutia* topically.

Resins, wood tar and turpentine oil (also called spirit of turpentine, and wood turpentine, made by distilling the resin), from pine trees were frequently mentioned in historical Greek texts and were used a great deal for skin complaints.

Mythology

According to Apollodorus and Plutarch, the pine tree was sacred to Poseidon, who had sacred pine groves at Corinth and Onchestos. Poseidon's son, Sinis Pityocamptes, the Pine-

Bender, was a Corinthian bandit who waylaid travellers passing through the Isthmus. He hid behind the pine trees, leaping out when a traveller passed by, catching the poor unfortunate victim and tying him to the top of a pine-tree, which he bent down until it touched the ground. When he released the tree it sprang up, catapulting the unfortunate captive into the air. Theseus encountered Sinis and killed him in the same manner. He then instituted the Isthmian Games to appease the ghost of Sinis and his father Poseidon. He crowned the victors of the games with wreaths of pine.

The Isthmian grove near Corinth was a pine tree grove. The pine tree was also sacred to Dionysos, whose devotees wielded pine or fir-cone tipped *thyrsoi* staffs.

Botanical Description

The Aleppo, *Pinus halepensis,* is a coastal pine which grows to a height of 15-25 m with a trunk diameter up to 60 cm. The bark is orange-red, thick and deeply fissured at the base of the trunk, and thin and flaky in the upper crown. Needles are pale green, usually 6-12 cm long and up to 0.1 cm wide, and are borne on silvery-grey branches, usually falling off after the second year. The Turkish pine (*Pinus brutia*) is another coastal pine, somewhat larger at 20-35 m, with a trunk diameter of up to a metre. The bark is orange-red, thickened and deeply fissured at the base of the trunk and thin and flaky in the upper crown. The young needles are smooth, 1.5-4 cm long, and continue to grow, in pairs, for 2-4 years. The adult needles stay on the tree for 1.5-2.5 years, with a persistent 1-1.5 cm sheath. It has edible seeds.

Local villagers tap pine resin from the Turkish pine. Resin seals the plant's wounds, kills insects and fungi and allows the plant to eliminate excess metabolites. Industry uses steam distillation to convert the resin into gum turpentine and gum rosin. Turpentine can be used as medicine, as well as for paint.

Unfortunately, Turkish pine forests are being cut down to make way for housing.

Healing Properties

Pine resin is antiseptic, expectorant, tonic, kills intestinal parasites, and is used externally against rheumatic pain, skin diseases and injuries, as well as to treat colds, coughs, flu, bronchitis and asthma. It is also used for inflammatory diseases and for healing ulcers in the digestive tract.

Chemical constituents

Pinus halepensis and *Pinus brutia* contain resins, gums and volatile oils. Gums mainly consist of polysaccharides and are rubbery and water soluble. The essential oils from *Pinus halepensis* and *Pinus brutia* contain mainly alpha pinene, beta pinene, caryophyllene, carene, camphene, limonene, ü-myrcene and myrtenol. Also, sabinene, cymene, turpinene, terpinolene, terpineol, linalol, fenchol, borneol, and many other compounds.

Research

In 1999 Digrak demonstrated that extracts of leaves, resins, barks, cones and fruits of *Pinus brutia* were anti-bacterial. Essential oils of the resin of *Pinus brutia* and *Pinus pinea* are anti-bacterial, phytotoxic, antioxidant and insecticidal, according to Ulukanli in 2014. In 2013 Cretu found that *Pinus brutia* extracts were effective free radical scavengers. In 2012 Süntar and team demonstrated *in vivo* that essential oils of *Pinus pinea* and *Pinus halepensis* were anti-inflammatory and wound healing. In 2003 Gülçin demonstrated that extract of turpentine (crude pine resin) from *Pinus nigra* ssp. *pallasiana* had a pain killing effect *in vivo*. The diterpene abietic acid is one of the major compounds in the non-volatile fraction of the resin of *P. brutia*. In 2001 Fernández demonstrated that abietic acid was anti-inflammatory *in vivo*. In another study in 2009 Ince and team demonstrated the *in vivo* anti-inflammatory activity of an extract from the bark of *P. brutia* in comparison to Pycnogenol®, a standardized bark extract of French maritime pine *Pinus maritima* Lam. At doses of 75 and 100 mg/kg *P. brutia* extract had a stronger anti-inflammatory effect than 10 mg/kg of indomethacin.

Gathering pine resin traditionally

Satil and Selvi describe the process of extracting and processing pine resin from *P. brutia* in Turkey. Local men make a V shaped cut into the trunk of a *P. brutia* tree; the resin flows out and begins to thicken within 5-10 minutes of air contact and they collect 50-200 g of resin per tree immediately.

The women boil the resin for 4-5 hours, stirring continually, until it is as thick as honey or jam. Then they strain it through a piece of cloth and collect it in a plate. Before it gets cold, they press it between the palms of their hands and put it into cold water to harden.

Local people mash the dried resin into powder, mix it with honey and take it to cure stomach and intestinal wounds, ulcers, and coughs. They chew pieces of resin to freshen their breath and clean their mouths. They make ointments from ground up resin. They boil the resin in water and use the resultant liquid on boils, heel cracks and injuries. Up until 10 or 15 years ago large numbers of people still harvested pine resin, but nowadays only a few still continue the practice. Pine resin has lost its value and *P brutia* forests are being cut down. Fires also threaten the forests.

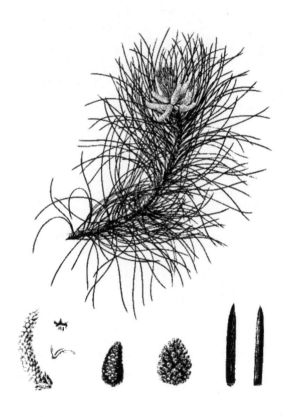

Pine Corsican and Pine stone *Pinus nigra laricio* and *Pinus pinea*

Mythology

The stone pine was sacred to Pan/Dionysos, who had sacred pine groves on Mount Mainalos. According to Lucian and Nonnus, the nymph Pitys fled the unwelcome advances of the God Pan and was transformed into a pine tree.

According to Antoninus Liberalis princess Dryope was tending her father's flocks on Mount Oeta, when she met the Hamadryads, who taught her to sing hymns to the gods and dance. On one occasion the Hamadryads took her into the forest and hid her. Maidens of the village spread the rumour that she had been abducted. The nymphs were angry and transformed the girls into pine trees.

According to the Homeric Hymns, the Oreiades were nymphs of the mountain peaks who were born and died with their native pines.

Botanical Description

The Corsican pine is a slender, conical, mountain growing tree which reaches a height of 20-55 m with horizontal branches. It is a subspecies of the European black pine. The bark is grey to yellow-brown, and is widely split by flaking fissures into scaly plates, becoming increasingly fissured with age. The needles are long, grouped in pairs and have a distinctive twist. Its large shining cones are always one-sided or oblique.

The stone pine is smaller, at 15-25 metres, has an umbrella-shaped crown, with horizontal upswept branches. It has orange/yellow/brown bark with deep longitudinal furrows and becomes scaly when mature. It produces edible pine nuts.

Healing Properties

Pinus pinea shares many of the healing properties of *Pinus brutia*. However, it is one of the 20 species of pine trees which produces pine nuts big enough to harvest. People use pine nuts traditionally to treat high blood pressure, to boost the immune system, or apply pine nut oil externally to treat a range of skin disorders. Pine nut oil contains pinolenic acid, a polyunsaturated fatty acid which stimulates cell proliferation, prevents hypertension, decreases blood fats and blood sugar, and inhibits allergic reactions. Pine nut oil is anti-bacterial, anti-fungal, anti-viral, antiseptic, anti-neuralgic, protects the liver, stimulates the secretion of bile, is diuretic, expectorant and lowers blood pressure.

Chemical constituents

Pine nuts contain minerals, especially potassium and phosphorus, as well as calcium, iron, magnesium, zinc, iron and manganese. Oleic and linoleic acids, including pinolenic acid, are the major unsaturated fatty acids, while palmitic, stearic and lignoceric acids are the main saturated ones. Pine nuts contain vitamins B1, B2 and C.

Research

In 2011 Amp found that when he fed pine nuts to rats their triglyceride levels fell, HDL cholesterol increased and LDL cholesterol levels fell. In 2017 Yang isolated 2 novel peptides from pine nut (*Pinus koraiensis*) meal protein. He demonstrated that they were antioxidant.

Unfortunately, people have been cutting down the stone pine forests all over the world, causing a scarcity of pine nuts. They have become so expensive that using them medicinally is almost impossible but we can still use them in our cooking, for example to make pesto.

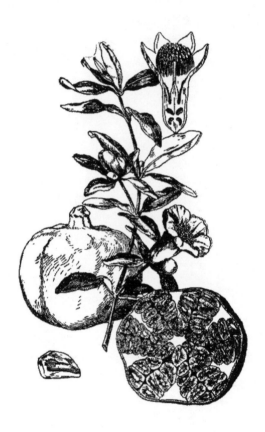

Pomegranate tree *Punica granatum*

Mythology

Damien Stone tells the story of the pomegranate, one of the oldest foods in the world, originating in Iran and domesticated during the Neolithic Revolution around 10,000 BCE. Its red juice is reminiscent of blood, it has a reputation for being aphrodisiac, is a symbol of fecundity and it embodies beauty, mystery and the female.

There was a mystery religion dating back to Mycenean times (ca. 1700 BCE,) devoted to Demeter and Persephone at Eleusis in Attica, supposedly where grain was first grown and Persephone returned to the Earth. The secret ceremonies of the mystery religion, promoting the idea of a pleasant existence after death for initiates, probably reenacted the myth of Persephone in the underworld, the pomegranate symbolising female fertility, and loss of virginity. On the other hand, Prakash in 1986 suggests that Persephone's eating pomegranate concerns women's use of birth control. Evidence for this came in the form of a cuneiform recipe from Aššur in which pomegranate seed, applied to wool, was placed in the vagina as a contraceptive, according to Campbell Thompson in 1949. In 2003 Pankaj Oudhia, reported that women in Chhattisgarh, India, ground pomegranate seeds into a powder, mixed in sesame oil, and placed the mixture in the vagina just after the menstrual cycle as a contraceptive. Pomegranates have a relatively high concentration of naturally occurring oestrogens and various parts, including seeds, roots, and fruit pulp contain various oestrogens including oestroil, oestrone and the powerful 17β-oestradiol. The modern contraceptive pill is based on a combination of oestrogen (to disrupt ovulation) and progestin (to prevent implantation).

Again, according to Damien Stone in 2017, the temple of Athena on top of the Acropolis housed a wooden statue of

Athena with a pomegranate in her right hand, representing the female battle, and a helmet in the left hand, representing the male battle. Athena is represented with pomegranate on several different ancient coins from Side (now in modern Turkey).

The word *side* is also ancient Greek for pomegranate, as well as being the name of Orion's wife. According to Apollodorus, Orion married Side, which also represents autumn ripening of the fruit. Side thought that she was as beautiful as Hera. Whoops! Always a mistake to compare yourself with Hera. Hera sent her to the Underworld forever, hence yet again the association between the underworld and the pomegranate. There may have been a secret cult around Hera and pomegranate connected with the Side myth. The blood red seeds of the pomegranate, symbol of female fertility, were sacred to Hera, who is also often represented holding a pomegranate.

The first pomegranate was said to have been created by Aphrodite from the blood of her dying mortal lover Adonis. The fruit was symbolic of the sexually powerful Aphrodite, who planted it on the island of Cyprus.

Cybele, ancient Phrygian mother of the gods, worshipped with orgiastic rites in the mountains of central and western Anatolia, holds a pomegranate in one hand and a mirror in the other. According to Apollodorus, in Phrygia, where Rhea was identified with Cybele, she purified Dionysus and taught him the mysteries.

When he was a baby Dionysus was torn up and eaten by Titans and from his blood a pomegranate tree grew. Certain ritual festivals banned eating pomegranates because they spring from the blood of Dionysus, although he was later reassembled and grew up into the lusty, wine drinking hero we know and love.

One day, when Agdistis was wreaking havoc among gods and men, Dionysus cleverly put wine into the water fountain where Agdistis came to drink, so that he got drunk and fell asleep. Dionysus tied his feet together and made a vine grow over his genitals. When Agdistis woke up and leapt to his feet his genitals were torn from his body by the vine and from the blood that spilled from his groin a pomegranate tree grew. A river nymph called Nana ate one of the pomegranates from the tree and the fruit impregnated her. She gave birth to Attis.

Dionysus seduced a maiden saying he would give her a crown. When she asked for her reward, he made her into a pomegranate tree.

Tantalus was punished by the gods and made to suffer eternally in the underworld, standing in a pool of water under a fruit tree with fruit just out of reach and the water receding before he could drink. Homer's Odyssey has him trying to reach a pomegranate.

Greek medicine prescribed pomegranate juice to stop menstrual bleeding.

Botanical Description

The pomegranate is a small deciduous tree or shrub which can grow up to 5-8 metres. The leaves are opposite, narrow, oblong 3-7 cm long and 2 cm broad. It has bright red, orange, or pink flowers, 3 cm diameter, with 4-5 petals. It produces a red fruit about the size of a large orange, rich in seeds and with a juicy red fruit pulp. The seeds are set close together in kaleidoscopic clusters, embedded in a yellow or white leathery pulp. The tree was cultivated in ancient orchards alongside the apple, pear, fig and olive.

Healing Properties

Pomegranates are anti-inflammatory, antioxidant, anti-bacterial and anti-fungal. They may help prevent cancer, lower blood pressure, alleviate arthritis, prevent heart disease, improve memory, improve athletic performance, prevent the onset of Alzheimers, help allay menopausal symptoms, prevent erectile dysfunction. Pomegranates have been used for thousands of years to treat sore throats, coughs, urinary infections, digestive disorders, skin disorders and arthritis. People use the peel, bark and leaves of pomegranate to calm the digestive system and prevent diarrhoea. They drink a tea made from the leaves to calm the stomach.

In the year 2000 the British Medical Journal chose the pomegranate as the logo for the Millennium Festival of Medicine. The pomegranate features in the heraldic crests of several medical institutions involved in the organisation of the festival. It has been revered through the ages for its medicinal properties.

Chemical constituents

Pomegranates contain minerals: calcium and phosphorus, vitamin C, tannins and several classes of flavonoids, including anthocyanins, flavan 3-ols and flavonols. They contain icosanoic-, linolenic-, punicic- and stearic- acids, phenolic compounds, such as gallic acid, chlorogenic acid, caffeic acid, catechin, phloridzin and quercetin. They contain a type of tannins, ellagitannins in the juice and peel: punicalagin and punicalin. Pomegranates also contain amino acids, such as proline, methionine and valine. Anthocyanins cause the red colour in the juice. Pomegranate seeds contain an oil, which is rich in punicic acid and the isoflavone, genistein, the phytoestrogen, coumestrol.

Research

The wonderful thing about pomegranates is that they contain a multitude of healing compounds which work together synergistically. David Weber from the University of California at Los Angeles Centre for Human Nutrition said:

"Our studies show that combinations of compounds act differently than single compounds in 2 ways. One is enhanced action. The other is that they are metabolised differently."

According to Newman in 2007 ellagitannin, a type of tannin found in pomegranate, is used by plastic surgeons to prevent skin flap death, due to its antioxidant activity. Pomegranate juice contains polyphenols which are highly antioxidant. Both the juice and peel contain catechins which are also highly antioxidant. All pomegranate flavonoids are antioxidant and anti-inflammatory.

Pomegranate tree bark and roots are rich sources of alkaloids, which people have used traditionally to treat worms in the human gastrointestinal tract.

According to Rettig in 2008, pomegranate fruit could delay the onset of prostate cancer, because it could inhibit cell growth and stimulate the immune system to remove cancer cells. In 2004 Albrecht and team investigated the effect of pomegranate seed oil, fermented juice polyphenols and pericarp polyphenols on human prostate cancer cell growth *in vivo*. They found that both the fruit extract, the oil, the juice polyphenols and the pericarp polyphenols had significant anti-tumour activity *in vivo*. In 2004 Mehta found that fermented pomegranate juice had double the anti-cancer effect of fresh pomegranate juice in human breast cancer cells lines. Pomegranate seed oil prevented the breast cancer cells from dividing and multiplying by 90 percent. In 2007 Khan and team found that pomegranate fruit extract inhibited human lung carcinoma cells. They suggested that pomegranate fruit extract could prevent lung cancer from developing.

In 2006 Adams reported the anti-inflammatory effects of pomegranate juice on signalling in human colon cancer cells. In 2008 Pacheco-Palencia demonstrated that pomegranate seed oil protects human cells from UVA and UVB damage *in vitro*.

Scientists have demonstrated the anti-atherosclerosis, blood pressure lowering and anti-inflammatory effects of pomegranate juice in the laboratory, according to Gil in 2000. Pomegranate juice helps to protect blood vessels from atherosclerosis, has anti-aging effects and is a potent antioxidant. Clinical studies have demonstrated that pomegranate juice reduces blood pressure, according to Stowe in 2011. But the studies were small and more larger studies need to be carried out.

Punicic acid, in pomegranate seed oil has an anti-cholesterol effect. In 2010 Mirmiran and team carried out a double-blind placebo-controlled clinical trial on 51 people with high cholesterol. They gave one group pomegranate seed oil twice a day for 4 weeks. Triglyceride levels fell in the group who took the pomegranate seed oil. It did not fall in the control group.

In 2009 Al-Zoreky found that pomegranate fruit peel was anti-bacterial and anti-fungal *in vitro*.

Conclusions

This is just a small amount of the research which scientists have carried out on the pomegranate tree and its fruit. There can be no doubt that eating pomegranates is good for you. Eating the whole fruit, including the seeds is even better than drinking the juice, since the seeds contain such wonderful healing compounds.

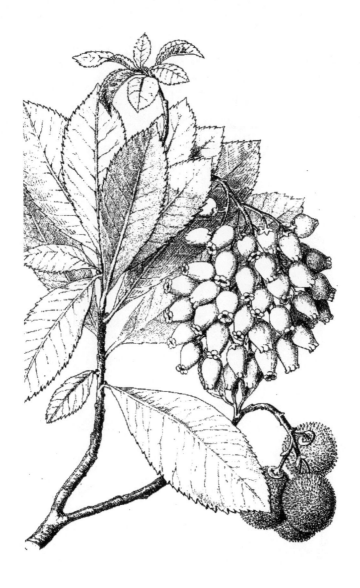

Strawberry tree Grecian *Arbutus andrachne* and *Arbutus unedo*

Mythology

The strawberry tree was sacred to Hermes who was nursed beneath one as an infant god, according to Pausanias. There was a sacred strawberry tree in his sanctuary at Tanagra. Apparently, Pliny the elder said *"unum tantum edo"*, meaning "I eat only one." From this the name *unedo* developed. No-one knows whether Pliny thought the fruit was so uninteresting that he only ate one, or whether it was so good that he could only eat one. The latter seems unlikely to me.

Botanical Description

Arbutus andrachne the Greek Strawberry tree, can reach a height of about 12 m. The smooth bark exfoliates during the summer, leaving a pistachio green layer, which changes to a beautiful orange brown. White bell-shaped flowers (resembling hot-air balloons) 0.4-0.6 cm diameter in panicles of 10-30 together, are produced in clusters (15–30 flowers) on red stems, and are nectar-scented. The leaves are dark green and glossy, 5-10 cm long and 2-3 cm broad with serrated edges. The edible fruit is a spectacular red berry 1-2 cm diameter, with a rough surface, which matures in 12 months, at the same time as the next flowering. Natural populations of *Arbutus unedo* are in danger due to deforestation, over-collecting and new construction on the coasts.

Healing Properties

The leaves, bark and root are astringent, antibiotic, anti-fungal and diuretic. Since they are antiseptic, they are used to treat cystitis and urethritis. Their astringent action makes them useful for treating diarrhoea and, like many other astringent plants, a gargle can be made for treating sore throats. Strawberry tree fruit has antioxidant and anti-cancer properties and strawberry tree honey is a rich source of healing compounds.

Chemical constituents

Arbutus berries contain plenty of vitamin C, malic and citric acid, as well as the minerals: potassium, calcium, phosphorus, magnesium and sodium. They are high in phenolics, including polyphenolic flavonoids, such as +catechin, −epicatechin and arbutin which are antioxidant. They are low in soluble sugars: fructose, glucose and sucrose. The berries have large amounts of carotenoid pigments: (All-*E*)-Violaxanthin and 9*Z*-violaxanthin are the major ones, responsible for the bright colour of the ripe fruits. In addition, the berries also contain other 5,6-epoxide carotenoids, such as (all-*E*)-neoxanthin, (9'*Z*)-neoxanthin (all-*E*)-antheraxanthin and lutein 5,6-epoxide, together with (all-*E*)-lutein, (all-*E*)-zeaxanthin and (all-*E*)-β-carotene. They also contain glycosides of anthocyanins, such as cyanidin-3-galactoside. Other antioxidants in this fruit were ellagic acid and its diglucoside derivative.

The tree bark contains compounds such as monotropein and unidoside.

Research

Numerous researchers, including Oliveira in 2009 and Fortalezas in 2010, have demonstrated that extracts of strawberry tree leaves are antioxidant and free radical scavenging *in vitro*. This is probably due to the large amount of phenolic compounds in the extracts.

In 2010 Tavares and team demonstrated that extracts of strawberry tree fruits and leaves were antioxidant and inhibited metallo-proteinases: which indicated that they could inhibit cancer cells from growing and spreading. In 2017 Afrin and team compared strawberry tree honey with Manuka honey as anti-cancer agents. They found that both types of honey stopped colon adenocarcinoma and metastatic cells from growing and spreading, probably because the honeys contained antioxidant compounds.

Several scientists have demonstrated that extracts of strawberry tree leaves are anti-bacterial. In 2017 Jurica and team found that the aqueous extract of the leaves, which is used traditionally to treat bladder infections, was strongly anti-bacterial *in vitro* against Enterococcus faecalis, a bacterium which often infects the bladder. In 2011 Orak and team found that strawberry tree leaves extract was anti-bacterial against Staphylococcus aureus and anti-fungal against 2 toxic moulds.

In 2018 Jurica and team found that high concentrations of arbutin, one of the strawberry tree flavonoids, did not damage human white blood cells or DNA. Nor did the extract.

Conclusions

This is one tree that we can grow in our gardens, if we have a garden because Strawberry trees will grow in a wide range of climates and soil types, though they do best in a nutrient-rich well-drained moisture-retentive soil in sun or semi-shade. Especially when young, they prefer a fairly sheltered position and dislikes cold drying winds. This is a very good tree to grow in towns because it tolerates industrial pollution. The white blossom and red fruit ripen in the winter and are delightfully decorative before you harvest the fruit to eat or make into jam.

Although there have not been many clinical trials to demonstrate the healing properties of the tree, people have been eating the fruit for centuries and it is perfectly safe. They have also been using the leaves, bark and root but there is insufficient evidence that these are safe.

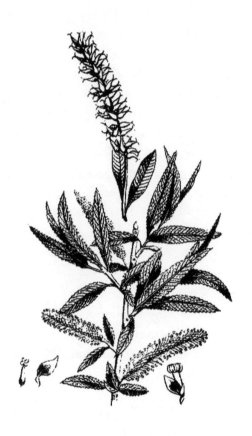

Willow white *Salix alba*

Mythology

The ancient Greek word for willow, helice, gave rise to Helicon, where the nine muses, priestesses of the moon goddess, lived. Helice, whose name suggests that she was a willow nymph or dryad, was Zeus's nurse during his infancy in Crete. The willow was sacred to Hekate, Circe, Hera and Persephone, all death aspects of the triple moon goddess, according to Robert Graves. Willow has been associated with grief and death, magic, feminine mysteries and the moon, since the dawn of time. Homer describes Persephone's sacred grove of willows and black poplars near the entrance of Hades, realm of the dead. The water-loving willow was sacred to the moon goddess, the giver of dew and moisture. People still use willow wands to find water.

According to Apollonius Rhodius, when Orpheus and the Argonauts walked into the garden of the Hesperides, the three nymphs wisely transformed themselves into trees to escape the ravages of the men. Erytheia became an elm, Hesperia poplar, and Aigle a willow tree.

People have probably been using willow as a painkiller since prehistoric times but the first records of its use date from 4000 BCE when the Assyrians used willow leaves to alleviate painful musculoskeletal joint pain and to bring down fevers, according to Jack in 1997. The Corpus Hippocraticum mentions willow to relieve pain in childbirth and for fever, according to Riddle in 1999. And according to Wells in 2003 Dioscorides mentions willow to reduce inflammation in his De Materia Medica Libri Quinque.

In 1763 Reverend Stone made the connection between the bitter taste of willow bark and Peruvian bark (Quinquona, source of quinine). Peruvian bark was already a well-known remedy for paroxysms, fever, malaria and rheumatism, so he suggested that since the two barks tasted the same, they might well have the same medicinal properties. He tested his hypothesis in a clinical trial lasting five years, using willow bark (S. alba) to treat paroxysms and fever from agues (malaria.) He observed that both types of bark had the same effects on his patients.

In the middle of the 18th century an English man accidentally chewed a twig from a willow tree, although it tasted horribly bitter, and discovered that his arthritic pain disappeared, according to Sutcliffe and Dunn in 1992.

People continued to use willow bark as a painkiller, until chemists isolated salicin from the bark, then synthesised salicylic acid, then acetyl salicylic acid from salicin, which became known as aspirin. After aspirin became one of the cheapest and most widely used drugs in the world, people stopped using willow bark.

Botanical Description

The white willow is a deciduous tree which grows to a height of 20-30 m with a rough greyish bark. The long thin leaves have saw-like edges and silky white hairs on both sides which give the tree a silvery sheen. Its flowers are catkins. Wicker baskets, shields and other items were made from its young, flexible stems.

Healing Properties

Willow bark is anti-inflammatory, anti-rheumatic and acts as a painkiller, so can be used for rheumatoid arthritis, rheumatism with inflammation and pain, and headaches. It will bring down a fever and reduce sweating, so can be used for influenza and the common cold. It is also antiseptic and the tannins in willow act as an astringent to reduce swelling. It will stop the itching of insect bites. It also acts as an anti-microbial. You can make a poultice by mashing up the bark or leaves, or you can make a strong tea, soak a piece of cloth in it and place it over an injury. Willow is the quintessential remedy for someone who is hot, inflamed, agitated, and stuck. It cools, eases rigidity, transforms harmful anger into discernment, and clears the way.

Chemical constituents

Willow bark contains salicylate, phenolic glycosides, tannins and flavonoids. The main constituents are listed in Caroll Newall's Herbal Medicines 1996. For an account of some to the research which has been carried out on willow please check my book "The Healing Power of Celtic Plants."

How to Use

Cut the young willow branches in the spring when the twigs are growing fast and the buds are swelling, then peel the bark with a knife. To make willow oil, cut the bark into small pieces and place them in a double boiler. Cover completely with an oil of your choice and heat very gently for several days, turning the oil on and off so that it does not boil. Strain with a piece of muslin cloth, then place the oil in a glass jar. It will last about a year in a cool dark place.

To dry willow bark and stem, place it in baskets, in a cool dark place. Make a tea with an ounce of dried bark in 2 pints of water. The tea is very bitter. Or powder the dried bark in a coffee grinder and fill capsules with it. Take 4-10 capsules per day.

To make willow tincture, place fresh cut bark and twigs in a glass jar and cover with vodka or brandy. Cover with a lid and let sit for at least 2 weeks. Shake the jar every few days and make sure the herb is under the liquid. Strain and bottle in a glass jar. If you are using dried willow bark, for every 30 g of dried willow, use 150 ml of vodka or brandy. Place in a jar and let sit for 2 weeks as above. The dosage is 30-60 drops. Tincture will last 7-9 years.

Contraindications

Anyone suffering from asthma, peptic ulcers, diabetes, gout, haemophilia, hypoprothrombinaemid, kidney or liver disease should be careful, just as they would with aspirin. Irritant effects of salicylate on the walls of the intestine are made worse by alcohol, barbiturates and oral sedatives. People taking anti-coagulants, methotrexate, metoclopramide, phenytoin, probenecid, spironolactone, and valepotrate should not take willow.

Part 3

The Plants and Flowers of Ancient Greek Myth

A vast range of flowering plants grow in Greece, from the Mediterranean flora of the coastlines, to the alpine flora of the mountains, with the addition of plants which came to the area from the east before the Aegean Sea existed. Now only 20% of Greece is still forested, due to the ravages of human occupation over the millennia, but more than 6,000 species of flowering plant and ferns have survived and 750 species of plants are unique to Greece, according to Hellmut Bauman.

Pliny the Elder recorded the works of more than 400 authors and 2,000 manuscripts concerned with various aspects of the natural environment in his Natural History, thus saving them from oblivion. Many other writers, such as Herodotus, Hesiod, Xenophon, Theocritus, Homer, Virgil, Ovid and Pausanias mention medicinal plants. Athenaeus in his learned Banquet describes the conversation at the dinner table between 23 learned men, who cover many subjects, including medicinal plants described in lost botanical works.

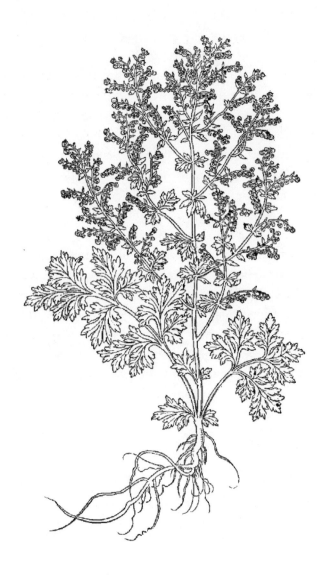

Artemisia, the "Mother Herb"

Artemisia is the name of a genus, composed of approximately 400 species of which more than 60 are used in traditional medicine, according to Wright in 2002. *Artemisia* is named after Artemis, virgin goddess of the hunt and the forest, one of the most popular goddesses in ancient times who protected women and wildlife. According to Manuela Dunn Mascetti in 1996, when Leto gave birth to Artemis, Leto suffered no pain; when Leto gave birth to Artemis's twin, Apollo, Artemis, miraculously already fully grown, helped her mother with a difficult birth. Midwives and "wise women" used various species of *Artemisia* for difficult births, which may explain why it was called the mother herb. According to Bently in 1995, there were many Artemis cults for women who were going through puberty, birth, motherhood and death.

Botanical Description of wormwood
Wormwood has a perennial root, from which firm leafy stems, covered in fine silky hairs, grow 60-75 cm high. It has whitish leaves also covered in hairs on both sides 7.5 cm long and 3.5 cm wide, cut deeply and repeatedly, the segments being narrow and blunt. The leaf-stalks are slightly winged at the margin. It has small, nearly globular flower-heads, arranged in erect, leafy panicles, with 3 leaves on the flower-stalks and the little flowers being pendulous and greenish-yellow.

Artemisia species that were used as medicine by the ancient Greeks include *Artemisia absinthium* or wormwood, *Artemisia abrotatum*, or southernwood, *Artemisia vulgaris* or mugwort. Wormwood has the most powerful properties, but all species of *Artemisia* kill internal parasites, which the ancients suffered from. Recent research by Caner in 2008 demonstrated that wormwood was effective against a number of digestive parasites.

Pliny said that *Artemisia*'s qualities were "specific to women." In Pseudo-Apuleius's Herbarius, he mentions that Diana, the Roman equivalent for Artemis, gave three types of *Artemisia* to Chiron the Centaur to use as medicine.

Dioscorides described why *Artemisia campestris* L. and *Artemisia arborescens* L. were especially good for women:

"When boiled, they are suitable to use in sitz baths for drawing the menstrual period, afterbirths, embryos/fetuses, for uterine closing and uterine inflammation, for breaking stones, and for retention of urine. The herb, when liberally plastered against the lower part of the abdomen, sets the menstrual period in motion. Its juice, triturated with myrrh and applied, draws from the uterus as many things as the sitz bath; the foliage is also given to drink in the amount of 3 drachmai to draw out the same."

Clearly Dioscorides is recommending *Artemisia* as an abortifacient and since *Artemisia species* are anti-inflammatory anti-bacterial, anti-viral, anti-coagulant, and stop bleeding, adding them to a sitz bath would have an additional healing effect.

In separate chapters Dioscorides recommends using southernwood (*A. abrotanon* L.) and absinthe (*A absinthium* L.) for menstrual problems. Today women take medicines containing *Artemisia species* for PMS, as they did in ancient Greece, but in ancient Greece women also took *Artemisia* when their menstrual periods were delayed, especially when they wanted to avoid pregnancy, according to John Riddle. The modern electronic guide to drugs, Drug Digest, specifies:

"Pregnant women should not take or use wormwood due to the risk of miscarriage. In animal studies, wormwood caused the muscles of the uterus to tighten, which could result in a miscarriage."

Dioscorides said of absinthe:

"It keeps mosquitoes away from the body when rubbed [on] with oil."

He added that putting absinthe in clothes chests keeps moths away; and adding it to ink keeps mice from eating the papyrus. According to Tan, Numerous modern science laboratory and clinical studies verify that compounds in absinthe, mugwort, and other *Artemisia species* are insecticidal against fleas, mites, and mosquitoes. Absinthe contains beta-thujone, which may contribute to the plant's insecticide and pesticide activities, according to Hélène Chiassonetal in 2001.

Soranus, a major authority on gynecology, prescribed absinthe to regenerate the body, and for chronic menstrual problems, such as lack of menstruation and heavy and painful menstruation. A Hippocratic work prescribed southernwood (*Artemisia abrotaton*) with pepper and honey in a lozenge for pneumonia and for pain caused by pleurisy.

Galen used southernwood and absinthe to treat internal parasites, stomachache, fevers and as a diuretic to expel internal poisons. He did warn that both plants were dangerous, especially absinthe which, he said, could cause coma.

Celsus recommended southernwood to treat quartan fever, i.e., malaria.

Today malaria continues to kill millions of children in the third world. So, the New York Times headline in February of 2008 was welcome news:

"There [are] reports of success with nets and the new medicine, artemisinin."

Artemisinin is derived from Chinese *Artemisia annua*. The ancient Greeks used other species of *Artemisia* as insecticides against mosquitoes and to reduce fever. Dioscorides said of absinthe:

"It keeps mosquitoes away from the body when rubbed [on] with oil."

Numerous modern science laboratory and clinical studies verify that wormwood, mugwort, and other *Artemisia* species contain insecticide compounds against fleas, mites, and mosquitoes.

By the 16th century wormwood was being added to a number of liqueurs. In 1792 Pierre Oridinaire, a French physician, fled the French Revolution to settle in Couvert, a Swiss village where he developed an absinthe alcohol, which he drank so much of that he died of its cumulative effects. His housekeeper started to make the absinthe liqueur, then gave the recipe to a Major Daniel-Henri Dubied, who passed it to Henri-Louis Pernod, his son-in-law. Pernod marketed the drink, and thus began the famous Pernod Fils Company in 1805.

During the Algerian war the French army doctors prescribed an absinthe alcoholic drink to treat malaria and intestinal parasites. The soldiers who were treated with the absinthe drink liked it so much that they began to drink it recreationally and brought it back with them to France. Like other forms of alcohol, it was intoxicating, but unlike other forms of alcohol it caused visual disturbances, unusual sensitivity to light and colour, mild euphoria, and a peculiarly clear-headed type of drunkenness. Absinthe contains alpha and beta-thujone which have mind-altering effects and can cause convulsions, vertigo, insomnia, nervousness, nausea, and tremors if taken in large enough quantities.

Ernest Hemingway's For Whom the Bells Toll has this conversation in the Spanish civil war between Robert Jordan, his central figure, and a gypsy about a bottle of absinthe:

"What drink is that?" the gypsy asked.

"A medicine," Robert Jordan said. "Do you want to taste it?"
"What is it for?"

"For everything," Robert Jordan said. "It cures everything. If you have anything wrong this will cure it."

"He [Robert Jordan looked forward to] being able to read and relax in the evening; of all things he had enjoyed and forgotten and that came back to him when he tasted the opaque, bitter, tongue-numbing, brain-warming, stomach-warming, idea-changing liquid alchemy. The gypsy made a face and handed the cup back.

"It smells of anise but it is bitter as gall," he said. "It is better to be sick than have that medicine." "That's wormwood," Robert Jordan told him. "In this, the real absinthe, there is wormwood. It's supposed to rot your brain out but I don't believe it. It only changes the ideas."

Hemingway was one of many writers and artists, including Edgar Degas, Gustave Moreau, Henri de Toulouse-Lautrec, Vincent van Gogh, Paul Gauguin, Pablo Picasso, Charles Baudelaire, Gustave Courbet, Paul Verlaine, Arthur Rimbaud, Oscar Wilde, Ernest Dowson, James Joyce, Amedeo Modigliani, Marcel Proust, Aleister Crowley, Erik Satie, Edgar Allan Poe, Lord Byron and Emile Zola, who were devoted to Absinthe liqueur. In 1859, Edouard Manet was the first of a long list of artists to paint absinthe drinkers, absinthe bottles, or both. Writers and artists believed that absinthe was the source of their inspiration. While touring America, Oscar Wilde said:

"Absinthe has a wonderful colour, green. A glass of absinthe is as poetical as anything in the world. What difference is there between a glass of absinthe and a sunset?"

Tiln Rekand and Ilmer Sulg carried out a study into the link between absinthe and creativity, focussing on the bursts of colours in Van Gogh's paintings. Van Gogh's mind produced the splendid images on canvas with yellow hues and halo effects, probably derived from a drug-distorted brain, according to Phillip E. M. Smith in 2006. What conversations he and Gauguin must have had when they drank absinthe together in Paris and Arles!

Today all Absinthe drinks contain less than 10 parts per million of thujone, the active compound from *Artemisia absinthum*, including the original Pernod Absinthe. St George Absinthe Verte is distilled in California, while Vieux Carre Absinthe is named after the New Orleans French Quarter. Absente Absinthe and La Fée Parisienne Absinthe are made in France. Sebor Absinthe is from Switzerland.

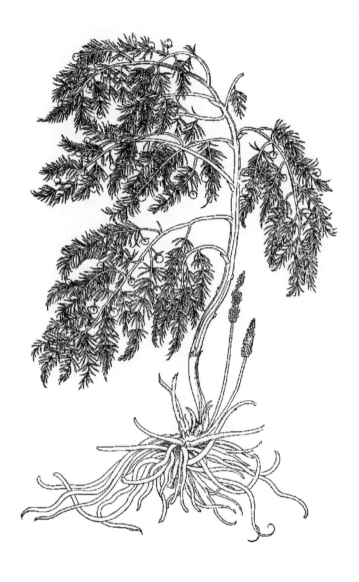

Asparagus *Asparagus acutifolius*

Mythology

Asparagus is sacred to Aphrodite. Perigune, daughter of the brigand Sinis, ran away when Theseus killed her father and hid on the isthmus of Corinth, behind an asparagus plant. Clearly it did not provide adequate cover, for Theseus found her and raped her, as was his habit. The Boeotians garlanded their fiancees with asparagus branches. Dioscorides and Theophrastus recommended eating the young shoots of wild asparagus.

Botanical Description

Asparagus acutifolius can grow up to a metre high with much branched stems and feathery foliage which consists in needle-like modified stems. It produces bell-shaped flowers in small greenish white clusters 4.5-5.5 mm long. Each plant bears either male or female flowers. The berries are 0.5-0.6 cm in diameter. It takes several years before one can harvest edible asparagus from the plants.

Healing Properties of Asparagus

Asparagus is anti-inflammatory, antioxidant, anti-fungal. People use asparagus traditionally to treat rheumatism. It helps detoxify the body and lower blood pressure, promote good cardiovascular health, healthy pregnancy, improved fertility, relief from the PMS, and improved bone health. It reduces urinary tract infections and blood cholesterol. It is also good for digestive health and has shown anticancer potential.

According to Alok in 2013, asparagus root is tonic, diuretic, galactagogue and ulcer healing, probably because it strengthens the lining of the gut. Ayurvedic doctors consider asparagus to be the queen of the herbs because it is a rejuvenating tonic for women. They believe that it is highly effective for treating problems related to female fertility and that it will increase longevity, immunity, vigour and vitality. They use it to treat nervous disorders, dyspepsia, inflammation and liver disease. They also use it to treat chronic fever. The root extract is anti-ulcer, antioxidant, anti-diarrhoeal, anti-diabetic and helps the immune system. It is also cooling, rejuvenating, carminative antiseptic and protects the nerves.

Chemical constituents

Asparagus contains high amounts of amino acids, including aspartic acid, which helps counteract excess ammonia, which can deplete the body of energy. Asparagus shoots contain thiophene, thiazole, aldehyde, ketone vanillin, acids and esters, as well as vitamins A, B1, B2, C, E, magnesium, phosphorus, calcium, iron and folic acid, amino acids, flavonoids, steroids, glycosides, according to Iqbal in 2017. It contains other antioxidants, such as glutathione, which helps promote a healthy immune system and liver. Asparagus contains steroidal saponins: shatavarins I-IV, which stimulate the immune system, are antioxidant, anti-bacterial, and protect the liver. It also contains asparagine A, a pyrrolizidine alkaloid, which is diuretic and breaks down oxalic and uric acid in the kidneys and muscles, so that they can be more easily eliminated. This helps to prevent the build-up of kidney stones. It contains diosgenin and quercetin.

Research

In 2017 Iqbal reviewed the therapeutic uses of Asparagus officinalis. High blood pressure is a growing problem and can lead to kidney and cardiovascular disease. Doctors prescribe angiotensin-converting enzyme (ACE) inhibitors to help dilate blood vessels and bring high blood pressure down. In 2013 Sanae found that when he fed asparagus to rats with high blood pressure, their blood pressure fell. He concluded that asparagus may contain compounds which inhibit ACE.

According to Sharma in 2000 saponins and fructans in asparagus have important anti-tumour activity and reduce the risk of constipation, diarrhoea, osteoporosis, obesity, cardiovascular disease, rheumatism and diabetes. Herbalists use the powdered dried asparagus roots to stimulate milk flow in breast feeding mothers. In 1967 Joglekar found that Asparagus racemosus root increased milk secretion in breast-feeding mothers. Thakur and Sharma reported that the roots are an effective remedy against diarrhoea and dysentery.

In 2006 Bhatnagar found that Asparagus racemosus root healed ulcers in rats. In 1997 De described a clinical trial in which 32 patients took the root powder and found that it healed their duodenal ulcers, probably, he concluded, because it strengthened the wall of the gut. In 2000 Mandal found that Asparagus racemosus root calmed the coughing of mice. In 1989 Regh demonstrated that asparagus had a normalising effect on damaged intestines of mice. In 2000 Mandal found that Asparagus racemosus root was anti-bacterial in vitro. In 2010 Zhu demonstrated that extracts of Asparagus officinalis protected the liver of mice who had been fed a high fat diet. In 2009 Gautam demonstrated that Asparagus racemosus root extract protected rats and mice from abdominal sepsis. It stimulated elements of the immune system to get rid of the infection at the same rate as metronidazole and gentamicin.

In 2013 Nishimura and team carried out a clinical trial giving the bottom stems of asparagus (the part that people usually throw away) to a group of people suffering from metabolic syndrome: high blood pressure, high blood sugar and high levels of fats in the blood. They gave powdered extract of the bottom stems and cladophylls (flat, green, leaflike structures) of asparagus (6g/day) to 28 healthy volunteers for 10 weeks. Their blood pressure and blood sugar went down, as well as their cholesterol.

Conclusions

Clearly the many species of asparagus contain powerful compounds with many important medicinal properties, but almost all the research has been carried out in the laboratory, with only a few clinical trials with low numbers of patients involved. So, I cannot recommend taking the root as a medicine. However, the young asparagus shoots that we love to eat are full of beneficial compounds. Unfortunately, the asparagus season is very short, but we should all eat as much of it as we can while it is available.

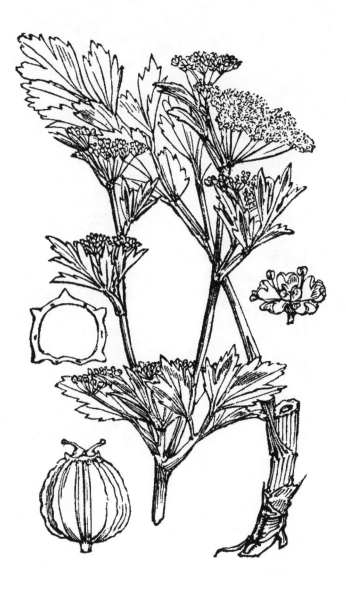

Celery and Parsley *Apium graveolens* and *Petroselinum sativum*

Mythology

The ancient Greeks dedicated celery to Hades, god of the underworld. They ate it at funeral meals, strewed it on graves and made it into wreaths for the dead. The Greek expression 'deisthai selinon' to need celery, meant that someone had just died. Pelikan said:

> *"Near Selinunt stood the temple of a chthonic underworld god called Apius to whom celery was dedicated."*

Celery and parsley were sacred to Zeus. Celery was also sacred to Poseidon. According to Apollodorus, Opheltes, the infant prince's nurse, lay him in a bed of wild celery while she gave directions to the 'Seven Against Thebes. A snake crept into the baby's crib and killed him. The warriors then founded the Nemean Games in his honour with a victor's wreath made from his celery death-bed. Thus, the wreath has the double symbolism of death and victory and victors of the Isthmian Games were crowned with celery, replacing the pine wreath.

The Greeks did not distinguish between parsley and celery. Wreaths of wild celery or parsley were worn by mourners at funerals and hung in tombs.

Botanical Description of Celery

Wild celery is a member of the Umbelliferae, a plant family that contains several poisonous species such as hemlock and giant hogweed, so do not go looking for wild celery, in case you pick the wrong plant, with fatal results.

Wild celery is a marshland plant with solid, grooved upright stems and can grow up to a metre tall. It has a shallow tap root system and the stem is branched, succulent and ridged. It has shiny branched leaves, each branch of which ends in 3 pointed leaflets, rather like daggers, 2-4.5 cm long. The leaves have short stalks or no stalks and are sheathed by a shiny petiole. In summer it produces small white flowers, in compound umbels, similar to those of cow parsley. Each tiny flower has 5 petals.

Healing Properties of Celery

Celery stalks and seed are powerfully anti-inflammatory. Celery stops the immune system from producing inflammatory nitric acid, reduces uric acid crystals in the body and decreases the production of inflammatory prostaglandins. Both the stalks and the seeds flush out uric acid crystals, are slightly diuretic and reduce the pain of gout, rheumatoid arthritis and osteoarthritis. Celery also prevents and cures ulcers of the digestive tract since it relaxes the walls of the gut as well as being anti-inflammatory. It is anti-bacterial, anti-fungal and even discourages some intestinal parasites. Celery reduces cholesterol, triglycerides and LDL (bad fats) and keeps the blood vessels clean and healthy.

The British Herbal Pharmacopoeia, 1983, records that celery seed is anti-rheumatic, sedative and a urinary antiseptic. It's recommended for rheumatism, arthritis, gout and inflammation of the urinary tract. It is potentiated by dandelion root, Taraxacum officinale. Celery seed is a mild diuretic and helps to flush away the uric acid crystals that build up around joints or collect in the kidneys to form kidney stones. It also helps to bring down high blood pressure. It is carminative, so eases stomach ache due to flatulence. It is a tonic, good for nervous conditions and helps to promote sleep. It lowers cholesterol, triglycerides and low-density lipoproteins (bad fats), so protects the blood vessels from plaque and helps to prevent cardiovascular disease. It is antioxidant and anti-inflammatory and helps to prevent gastric ulcers. It is anti-fungal.

For a full description of the chemical constituents and scientific research into the healing properties of celery, please consult my book: "Healing Plants of the Celtic Druids."

How to Use

Above all eat raw, organic celery leaves and stem as often as possible to allay the pain of rheumatoid arthritis, to prevent ulcers and to keep your blood vessels clear of plaque. Eat plenty of celery to keep sperm healthy if you are a man, to prevent menopausal symptoms and PMS is you are a woman. You should consult a trained herbalist for treatment with celery seed for kidney stones, rheumatism, rheumatoid arthritis and osteoarthritis.

Contraindications

Avoid celery seed during pregnancy and breastfeeding. People taking thyroxine should not take celery seed, since it inhibits thyroxine uptake. Celery does not cause sensitivity to sunlight by itself but it can cause increased risk of sunburn in people who take prescription ACE inhibitors to control high blood pressure. Many people are allergic to celery so since 2005 the Food Standards Agency has listed it as one of the 12 foods which must be shown clearly on the ingredient list of pre-packed food. Anyone with an allergy to birch pollen, nut or kiwi fruit should not take celery seed.

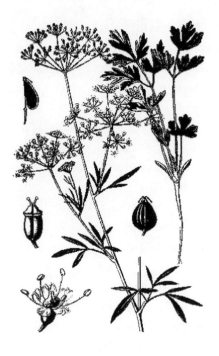

Botanical Description of Parsley

Parsley is a bright green hairless biennial plant. In the first year it forms a rosette of flat, compound pinnate leaves and a tap root. In the second year it grows a flowering stem up to a metre tall with sparse leaves and umbels of white flowers.

Healing Properties of Parsley

Parsley is anti-bacterial, anti-fungal, anti-coagulant, diuretic, antioxidant and oestrogenic. It contains compounds which lower blood sugar and blood pressure. It contains plenty of vitamin C and iron. It purifies the blood, dissolves sticky deposits and helps to maintain the elasticity of the blood vessels. It helps to dissolve small kidney stones and gallstones, stimulates the bowel and the adrenals. People take parsley tea to treat urinary infections, fluid retention, flu and colds, to lessen asthma attacks, to treat anaemia and to stimulate the liver. According to Alireza in 2012 traditional medicine has used parsley to cure allergy, autoimmune diseases and chronic inflammatory disorders. In Morocco traditional healers use parsley to treat high blood pressure, according to Ziyyat in 1997.

Chemical constituents

Parsley contains phenolic compounds, coumarins, furano-coumarins, vitamin C and E, carotenoids, flavonoids: quercetin apigenin, apiin and luteolin, which are antioxidant; and terpenes. There is a volatile oil in parsley which contains a complex collection of compounds, including alpha-pinene, beta-myrcene, alpha-phellandrene, mentha, apiol, myristicin and many other compounds. Apigenin is a flavone in parsley with antioxidant activity *in vitro*, according to Fraga et al in 1987. Parsley seed contains apiin, a glycoside, and volatile oil.

Research

According to Marczal in 1997 parsley seeds contain high quantities of essential oil and are diuretic. Since diuretics increase the flow of urine, they help the body to wash out bacteria as well as kidney stones. In 1999 Nielsen found that parsley had an antioxidant effect which, according to Hempel in 1999 was due to the flavonoids in it, including apiin, luteolin, apigenin, vitamin C and E. According to Vora in 2009, parsley protects the mitochondria of mice from oxidative damage, possibly due to the presence of flavonoids. Mitochondria are responsible for creating energy in our cells, so protecting them will ensure that we have a good supply of energy. In 2006 Ozsoy found that parsley reduced blood sugar in rats and this was due, according to Pino in 1997, to terpenoids. According to Anand in 1981 flavonoid glucosides and coumarins in parsley seeds reduce blood sugar. In 2004 Bolkent found that parsley protected the liver of diabetic rats from damage. Apigenin is anti-inflammatory according to Lee in 1993. In 2002 Manthey found that apigenin inhibited lung, colon, breast, prostate, brain and skin cancer cells *in vitro*. According to Ozturk in 1991 parsley is anti-coagulant, reduces fats in the blood, protects the liver and lowers blood pressure. In 2011 Chaves found that extracts of parsley prevented platelets from sticking together. Platelets stick together to form a scab over a wound, but they can also form plaques in the blood vessels, which leads to atherosclerosis (hardening of the arteries). In 2007 Jeong demonstrated *in vitro* that apigenin stops monocytes (a type of immune cell) from sticking to LDL cholesterol, one of the first stages of atherosclerosis. In 2007 Ueda demonstrated that flavonoids were anti-inflammatory *in vivo,* yet another reason why parsley might prevent atherosclerosis. Janssen reported in 1998 that the flavonoids quercetin and apigenin were responsible for this effect. In 2006 Wong and Kitts found that the phenolic part of a parsley extract was antioxidant and anti-bacterial. Parsley is also anti-fungal.

After the menopause many women suffer from insufficient oestrogen, which can lead to osteoporosis and high blood cholesterol. Kitagawa in 1976 found that extracts of parsley acted like oestrogen, as powerfully as soybean isoflavone glucoside.

There have been very few clinical trials with parsley, but it contains numerous active compounds and people have been using it in the kitchen and as medicine for many centuries.

How to use

Parsley is best eaten raw, added to salads as well as any other dish. Add a couple of spoonful's of chopped parsley to your meal to enjoy its health benefits. In countries where traditional healers prescribe parsley as a medicine, they use far higher quantities, but there is insufficient evidence of the safety of high doses, so we should not self-prescribe.

Contraindications

Women should be careful not to eat too much parsley because it can interfere with the menstrual cycle. Some people are allergic to parsley. Parsley seed oil should always be diluted in a carrier oil, such as almond oil. It can cause the skin to become extra sensitive to the sun and develop a rash. Pregnant women should be careful not to consume too much parsley as large amounts will cause them to miscarry. There is some evidence that taking a herbal combination of An-Tai-Yin and parsley during the first three months of pregnancy increases the risk of birth defects. It is probably best not to take large amounts of parsley while breastfeeding. People with bleeding disorders should avoid large amounts of parsley because it could increase the risk of bleeding. Diabetics should be careful not to take too much parsley because it can lower blood sugar. Don't take large amounts of parsley if you have a kidney disease. Stop taking parsley two weeks before surgery.

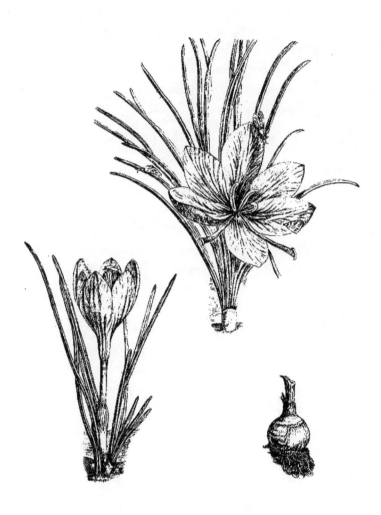

Crocus saffron *Crocus sativus*

Mythology

According to Ovid and Pliny, the god Hermes loved a boy called Krokos (Crocus). One day, as they were playing, Hermes accidentally hit Krokos on the head and killed him. Grief-stricken Hermes transformed him into a saffron flower, whose red stigmata looked like his spilt blood. Alternatively, three blood drops from his head fell onto the flower of the plant and the stigmata were created. Either way the plant became known as Krokos (Crocus,) and saffron became sacred to Hermes. According to other sources Krokos was metamorphosed into the flower after his love, the Nymph Smilax, died.

The Homeric hymns tell the tale of the goddess Persephone and her companion Nymphs, who were gathering rose, crocus, violet, iris, lily and larkspur in a springtime meadow when Hades burst out of the earth and dragged her down to his domain.

According to Hesiod, Zeus saw the Phoenician princess Europa in a meadow, where she was picking flowers. He transformed himself into a bull and breathed a crocus from his mouth to attract her. As she came near, he grabbed her and carried her away.

Botanical Description

There are about 100 species of crocus, most of which are native to the Mediterranean region. The plants start to grow after the first autumn rains and continue until late spring after which they survive the summer drought below ground. Numerous greyish green leaves sprout up, either together with the flowers, or shortly after. The flowers of Crocus sativus are pale pinkish lilac to deep lilac-blue, usually with slightly darker veins. The outer tube of the flower is 4-7 cm long, white, lilac or purplish

191

and divides into 1-9 segments, or petals, 2.5-5 cm long and 5-8 cm wide. Inside the flower are filaments 0.2-0.5 cm long and yellow anthers 0.9-2 cm long. The style is divided into 3 red branches, each branch 0.3-1.5 cm long, thin and tapering gradually to the expanded tip. These red styles are dried out to produce the drug saffron.

Saffron, the dried red styles, or stigmata, of Crocus sativus is the most expensive spice in the world. People use it to flavour and colour food. It is also being investigated as an anti-cancer drug, but since only 6 kg can be harvested from a hectare of land this is too little to be of much use. Scientists hope to increase the amounts of its active compounds by growing them in in vitro tissue cultures.

Healing Properties of Crocus
Saffron relieves tension, anxiety, depression, PMS, insomnia and is anti-spasmodic, expectorant and is reputed to be aphrodisiac. It may reduce the risk of heart disease and lower blood sugar levels and it may help prevent macular degeneration. It might improve the memory of people with Alzheimer's disease. According to Bhargavak in 2011, traditional healers in Iran use saffron to treat depression, stomach ache and insomnia. They apply a paste containing saffron to the skin to treat acne.

Chemical constituents
Saffron contains carotenoids: crocin and crocetin; pricrocrocin, and safranal. Crocus petals contain kaempferol.

Research
Most of the research into the healing properties of saffron have been carried out in the laboratory, often focussing on single compounds from the plant. Crocin from saffron is highly antioxidant according to Assimopoulou in 2005. In 2006 Papandreou demonstrated that crocin reduced blood fats in rats.

In 1999 Xuan demonstrated that crocin and analogues of crocin increased blood flow to the retina and choroid, and helped the retina to recover. This could be used to prevent ischaemic retinopathy and macular degeneration which sometimes occur in elderly people. In 2000 Abe demonstrated that saffron extract improves learning behaviour in mice. He concluded that crocin may be the active compound responsible for this effect. Saffron extract or its active compounds may be useful for treating memory loss due to degeneration of the nerves in the brain.

In 2004 Ochiai demonstrated that crocetin from saffron protects the heart of rats, due to its powerful antioxidant effect. In 2006 Xi demonstrated that crocetin had anti-diabetic effect in rats and prevented insulin sensitivity. In 2005 Ahmad found that crocetin protected rats' brains from damage caused by dopamine. Dopamine is used to treat Parkinson's.

In 2005 Hosseinzadeh demonstrated that safranal from crocus had anticonvulsant effect in mice. In 2006 Boskabady demonstrated that crocus has a relaxing effect on guinea pig smooth muscle. He suggested that it could be used to treat respiratory disorders such as asthma. In 2004 Wilburn and team found that extract of Crocus sativus petals reduced blood pressure in rats.

There have been a few small clinical trials. In 2004 Akhondzadeh and team carried out a double-blind clinical trial, comparing saffron to imipramine on a group of adult patients with mild to moderate depression. Patients were randomly assigned capsules of saffron 30mg/day or imipramine 100mg/day. Saffron at this dosage was as effective as imipramine. In 2005 Noorbala and team also carried out a double blind randomised clinical trial, this time comparing saffron extract with fluoxetine for treating mild to moderate depression. 40 patients were randomly assigned capsules of saffron 30mg/day or fluoxetine 20 mg/day. Saffron was as effective as fluoxetine. In 1998 Verma gave 50 mg saffron dissolved in 100 ml milk twice a day to 20 people. They measured lipoprotein oxidation susceptibility (LOS) at the beginning of the trial and at the end. They found that LOS levels fell, which indicated that the saffron was acting as an antioxidant. In 2005 Chatterjee carried out a randomised controlled clinical trial, giving an itch cream containing Crocus sativus at a concentration of 0.025% v/w to patients suffering from various skin conditions, including dermatitis and Ichthyosis vulgaris. It helped to reduce the itching.

How to use

Buy the threads of saffron, not the powder, and soak them in hot (not boiling) water, for a few hours, or overnight, then add the soak water to your recipes. Saffron powder may be adulterated with all kinds of substances, such as beet, red-dyed silk fibres, turmeric, paprika etc. Saffron goes well with rice dishes, such as paella, risotto etc. Or take as a dietary supplement.

Dosage

30 mg/day

Contraindications

People who are allergic to Olea and Salsa plant species may also be allergic to saffron. High doses: 5g or more, are toxic. Pregnant women should not take doses larger than the amount used in food. People suffering from bipolar disorder should avoid taking saffron since it may trigger excitability. Always buy the strands from a reputable brand or shop to make sure that you get the real thing.

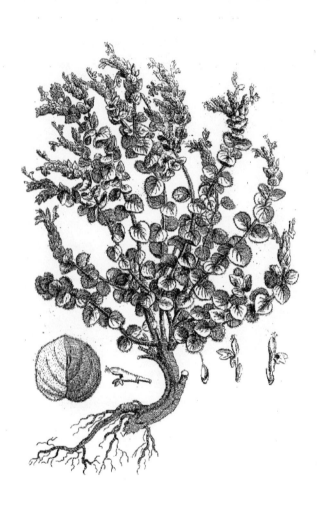

Dittany *Origanum dictamnus*

People in Crete have been using dittany as a healing herb since prehistoric times. When the Knossos palace near Heraklion was excavated archeologists found seeds of Origanum dictamnus, Artemisia absinthium, Salvia triloba and other aromatic plants, dating back to the Minoan era (27th-15th century BCE), according to Diapoulis in 1980. This, he suggested, proves the existence of ancient laboratories, which produced essences and cosmetics using aromatic plants. Between 1700 and 1450 BCE, the Minoan civilisation decorated their pottery and murals with pictures of plants for the first time. Some of the pictures are so realistic that the species of plant, including dittany, can be identified.

Mythology

Pliny says:

> *"The plant called* dictamnon *grows in no other place but on the island of Crete."*

Originally dittany was dedicated to the ancient Cretan goddess Diktynna. Minos, king of the Minoan civilisation, lusted after her and chased her. She ran away and threw herself into the sea, near the cape of Psakos (modern Spatha) but she was saved by the fishing-nets of local fishermen, so they called her Diktynna from the Greek word dikti for net. Diktynna was later matched with Artemis and became Artemis-Dictynna, goddess of the forest, the hunt, the mountains, springs and rivers. Both the plant and the goddess assisted childbirth and treated gynaecological disorders.

However, Skrubis in 1979 suggested that the species name, dictamos may also derive from Dicti, the Cretan mountain where Zeus was raised by the goat Amalthia and the Greek word *thamnos*, meaning shrub.

Homer reported that a bitter root was used to cure gastric ulcers and bleeding and in 1902 Berendes identified Homer's bitter root as dittany.

Hippocrates is reputed to have used dittany to cure gastric complaints, tuberculosis and in poultices on wounds. Aristotle and Theophrastus, according to Thanos in 1994, Dioscorides, according to Berendes in 1902, Galen and Plutarch, according to Liolios in 2010, all state that the wild goats of Mount Ida on Crete used to eat dittany shoots to heal their wounds when struck by poisoned arrows. This tradition passed to the Romans and famous Latin writers such as Cicero and Virgil attributed the healing of the Trojan hero Aeneas' wounds to Dittany of Crete, according to Hunt in 2005. Both Artemis and dittany could magically cure arrow wounds, which explains why Artemis is often represented with a crown of dittany on her head, according to Skoula and Kamenopoulos in 1997. Some ancient vernacular names like veloulko or velotoko (velos, arrow) probably refer to the plant's ability to heal arrow wounds, according to Gennadios in 1914, a very important property at a time when men were constantly fighting and wounding each other.

Other vernacular Greek names include stomachohorto, from Greek stomachos, stomach, referring to its stomach ache healing properties, and horto, herb, according to Plimakis in 1997. Kephalohorto means herb for the head, from the Greek kephali, head; stamatohorto means herb to stop bleeding, from Greek stamato, to stop; livanohorto means sweet smelling herb, from Greek livani, incense. Maliarohorto means hairy herb, from Greek maliaros, hairy, and gerondas means old man: since the dittany's leaves are covered in dense white hairs, according to Skoula and Kamenopoulos in 1997. All of which indicates the high repute in which this plant was held.

Theophrastus says dittany was used during cases of

prolonged labour. The Hippocratic Corpus also mentions using it for lung problems and in labour and calls the herb okytokion, from the words okys, meaning rapid and tokos, to give birth.

Botanical Description

Dittany is a perennial bushy sub shrub with aromatic foliage, which grows inside fissures of calcareous cliffs, usually in shadowy places from 300 m up to 1,500 m altitude, high up on the rocky slopes of the mountains of Crete. Today wild dittany is rare and hard to find because excessive harvesting has reduced it almost to extinction. It is now protected by the Berne Convention and included as a Priority Species in Annexes II and IV of the European Directive 92/43/EEC Habitats Directive. However, people have been cultivating it since the 1920s, so although picking wild dittany is prohibited (and extremely dangerous!) there are plentiful supplies of the cultivated plant.

It grows 20-30 cm high with many branches. Its stems are yellow or purplish brown and covered in branching hairs about 2 cm long. There are up to 15 pairs of roundish to oval leaves on each stem, the lower ones with short stems. The leaves are 1.5 cm long and 1.5 cm wide with raised veins on the underside. They are thin, whitish green, and covered in 0.2 cm long wooly hairs on both sides with up to 600 inconspicuous glands per square cm. What appear to be flowers are actually 16 cm long spikes of overlapping greenish or deep pink bracts, with 8 pairs of bracts per spike, roundish to ovate and 0.7 cm wide, which mature to showy reddish-purple as the seeds begin to form. 2 tiny flowers protrude from each spike of bracts with 0.35 - 0.5 cm long sepals and one lip. The flowers are 1.1cm long and 2 lipped, pink with stamens up to 1.4 cm long. Styles 1.8 cm long, protrude between the filaments of the stamens.

Healing Properties of Dittany

Dittany is a powerful healing and restorative herb. It was considered a panacea in ancient Greece and was used to treat stomach disorders, gastric ulcers, to cure the spleen, to treat rheumatism and to facilitate childbirth. It stimulates fresh skin to grow over a wound. In Greece it is traditionally made into an infusion called vrastari.

In 2013 the European Medicines Agency Committee on Herbal Medicinal Products (HMPC) concluded that dittany of Crete can be used as a tea to relieve cough, cold, stomach and digestive disorders. Dressings soaked in dittany infusion can also be applied to the skin to relieve inflammations and bruises. Although there have not been any clinical trials to support the use of dittany, they agreed that the experimental studies which had been carried out indicated that dittany is effective and safe with no side effects.

Chemical constituents

Dittany contains essential oils rich in volatile compounds such as carvacrol, terpinene, thymol and p-cymene, according to Liolios in 2010, which are anti-microbial, antioxidant and anti-ulcer. It also contains high concentrations of polyphenolic compounds, such as rosmarinic acid and salvianolic acid according to Exarchou in 2013; coumarins, triterpenes, tocopherols and sterols, according to Komaitis in1988; flavonoids including, apigenin, kaempferol and quercetin, which are anti-bacterial and anti-fungal, according to Chatzopoulou in 1985; and fatty acids, according to Revinthi-Moraiti et al 1985.

Research

In 2010 Liolios reviewed the research that had been carried out on dittany, which demonstrated that it was effective against sore throat, cough and gastric ulcer. These are just a few of the scientists who have carried out research on dittany: in 2003

Couladis found that extracts of dittany were as powerfully antioxidant as alpha tocopherol (Vitamin E); In 2013 Exarchou demonstrated that the depsides in dittany extract were responsible for the antioxidant effect. In 1982 Bazaios stated that it was diuretic and digestive and emmenagogue. In 1997 Skoula and Kamenopoulos demonstrated the anti-spasmodic effect of dittany and in 1996 Sivropoulou demonstrated that the essential oil of *Origanum dictamnus* was anti-bacterial and that the strongest anti-bacterial compounds in the oil were carvacrol and thymol. In 2001 Karanika found that aqueous extracts of *Origanum dictamnus* stopped yeast from growing. In 1997 Skoula and Kamenopoulos demonstrated that it was anthelmintic. All this research was carried out in the laboratory.

How to Use

Make a dittany tea to relieve tension headaches, as a relaxant and to relieve indigestion, stomach cramps and bloating. Take it to heal gastric ulcers and to relieve colds and coughs. Make a poultice with dittany to apply to wounds and bruises. Dittany skin cream is purifying, anti-aging and soothing. Dittany shampoo will strengthen your hair and scalp.

Dosage

Daily dose: 4.5 g
Herbal tea: 1.5–7 g of dried herb in 150 ml of boiling water. Allow to steep for 2–4 minutes. Take 3 times daily.

Make an infusion with 30–75 g of herb in one litre of water to use on the skin. Soak a dressing in the infusion and apply to the affected area, 2 to 5 times daily.

Contraindications

Pregnant and breastfeeding women should avoid dittany. Some people are allergic to it. Don't give dittany to children or adolescents under 18 years.

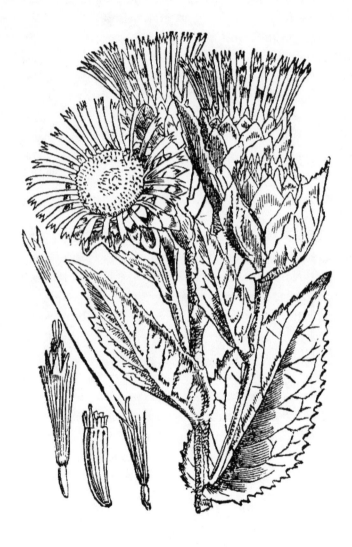

Elecampane *Inula helenium*

Theophrastus referred to elecampane as Chiron's all heal. Elecampane grows in the wooded valleys of Thessaly and people have been using it as medicine since the time of Hippocrates. Asclepius referred to elecampane as Chiron's root.

Mythology

After the fall of Troy, the seafarer Canapus took Helen and Menelaus to Egypt. Helen wept when he died and Helenium sprang from her tears. Another myth tells the story of Helen with arms full of elecampane when Paris stole her away to Phrygia. Yet another that Helen first used it against venomous bites and lastly, that it took the name from the island Helena, where the best plants grew.

Botanical Description

Elecampane is one of the tallest members of the Compositae family. It is perennial and grows up to 1.5 metres, with deeply furrowed, thick, hairy stems which branch near the top. At the base of the stalks, it produces a rosette of enormous, oval, pointed leaves on long stalks, from 30-45 cm long and 10 cm broad in the middle, velvety underneath, with toothed edges. The leaves on the stem become shorter and relatively broader and clasp the stem. It produces very large bright yellow flowers, almost as large as sunflowers: up to 10 cm in diameter, on long stalks. The broad bracts of the leafy involucre under the head are velvety. The root is large and succulent, spindle shaped, branching, brown and aromatic.

Elecampane is easy to grow from seed. It will even grow between the cracks of pathways.

Healing Properties

Elecampane root is an aromatic stimulant and tonic. It is also diuretic, diaphoretic, expectorant, antiseptic, astringent and gently stimulant. Herbalists use elecampane for coughs, influenza, bronchitis and asthma. When a person is suffering from bronchitis the lining of the bronchial tubes becomes swollen and red, making it harder to breathe. The inulin in the root coats and soothes the lining of the throat which results in a reflex soothing effect on the bronchi. It acts as an expectorant to make a dry, irritating cough productive and helps to clear congestion from the lungs and bronchi. Since elecampane is bitter it stimulates the flow of bile, the appetite and digestion. The British Herbal Medicine Association states that the sesquiterpene lactones in the roots of elecampane are powerfully antiseptic, healing and relaxant.

Chemical Constituents

For a full description of the chemical constituents and research that has been carried out on Elecampane see my book: "Healing Plants of the Celtic Druids."

How to Use

Elecampane root is powerful at clearing infections from the lungs. Take 10-15 drops of the tincture several times a day, to treat cough, bronchitis and asthma, but increase the dose and take it as much as 6 times a day if the infection is acute. Only take elecampane to treat an active infection. It will help relax the trachea and bronchi, make a dry cough productive and soothe the throat. Combine elecampane root decoction or tincture with mullein to make a cough mixture or take a cough syrup or lozenges containing elecampane. Also use it to aid digestion, to relieve night sweats and to lift your spirits.

Contraindications

Elecampane is generally safe and well-tolerated as long as it is used in moderation, especially for the young or elderly. Excessive doses will upset the stomach. Do not take during pregnancy or breastfeeding. People with diabetes or heart problems should not take elecampane. Large doses can cause diarrhoea and vomiting. People who are allergic to Asteraceae family pollen (chrysanthemum, chamomile, ragweed, daisy) may be allergic to elecampane.

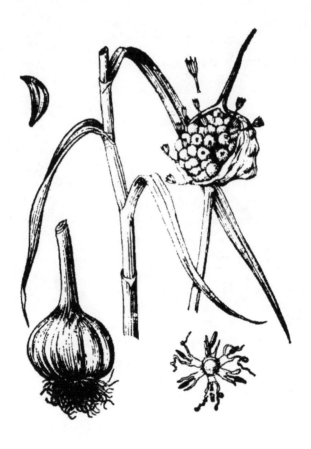

Garlic *Allium sativum*

Garlic originated somewhere in central Asia, and people have been using it as a medicine since prehistoric times, from West Europe to China. Aristophanes saw it as a sign of physical strength, but the gods hated the smell of it, so no one entered a temple smelling of garlic. Dioscorides talks about a wild garlic called ophioscordon (serpents' garlic). This could have been Allium ursinum. He said it was laxative and would drive out tapeworms. He prescribed garlic mixed with honey to treat leprosy, skin blemishes and dandruff. He also recommended garlic for colic relief, for regulating the menstrual cycle and against seasickness.

Ashurbanipal, the last great tsar of Assyria, described how physicians used garlic to bring down body temperature, as a remedy against constipation and muscle inflammation and to kill intestinal parasites. The Hippocratic Corpus also mentions that garlic kills intestinal parasites.

The Egyptians fed garlic to their slaves to keep them strong, while giving them less food. Herodotus wrote:

"Inscriptions on the plates of the Egyptian pyramids tell us how much their builders used the garlic for this vegetable, 1600 talents of silver were spent" (approximately 30 million dollars).

From Egypt garlic spread round the shores of the Mediterranean to Palestine, Greece and ancient Rome. Archeologists excavating Knossos Palace on Crete found garlic bulbs dating from 1850–1400 BCE according to Petrovska in 2010. Early Greek army leaders fed their army with garlic before major battles. According to Theophrastus (370–285 BCE), the Greeks offered garlic bulbs to their gods, which seems strange since other sources state that the gods hated the smell of it. In the Middle Ages, people in Europe used garlic to prevent them from catching the plague. In 1720 four thieves in Marseilles were offered freedom in exchange for them burying the plague dead. They made a mixture of chopped garlic and wine, which they drank all day while burying the dead and survived the plague.

Botanical Description

Garlic is a member of the lily family, or Liliaceae, with long, smooth, flat leaves 0.8 cm wide. The greenish, whitish flowers are at the end of a stalk rising straight up from the bulb, grouped together in a globular head, or umbel, with an enclosing leaf, and among them are small bulbils. Garlic has a compound bulb, consisting of numerous cloves, which fit together between membraneous scales, enclosed within a whitish skin.

Properties

Garlic is powerfully anti-bacterial, anti-viral, antioxidant and anti-parasitic. It protects from LDL cholesterol (bad fats.) It decreases the concentration of triglycerides and cholesterol in blood and prevents them from sticking to the sides of the blood vessels, so reducing the risk of atherosclerosis and heart diseases. Since humans excrete allicin partly through the lungs, herbalists use garlic to treat respiratory tract diseases.

Chemical constituents

Garlic contains sulphur glycosides, which give it its characteristic smell. It contains alicin, quercetin, cellulose, amino acids, lipids, etheric oil, complex fructosans (carbohydrates), steroid saponosides, organic acids, vitamins C, A, and B complex, enzymes etc. It contains minerals: manganese, potassium, calcium, phosphorous, magnesium, selenium, germanium, sodium, iron, zinc and copper. For a full account of the chemical compounds in garlic please consult my book "Healing Plants of the Celtic Druids."

Research

There has been masses of research into the healing properties of garlic and individual garlic compounds. For a full description of this research please consult my book "Healing Plants of the Celtic Druids." Garlic prevents thrombosis and blood clots, protects against free radicals, prevents cancer cells from growing and spreading and brings down high blood pressure.

Today, many pharmacopoeias throughout the world, including the European Pharmacopoeia, the United States Pharmacopoeia and the British Pharmacopoeia, prescribe garlic as well as garlic preparations.

How to Use

The German Commission E recommends that people with high levels of cholesterol should eat fresh garlic or take it as a supplement to prevent hardening of the arteries. People who suffer from gastric diseases and people who produce too much hydrochloric acid cannot tolerate garlic. Therefore, many manufacturers produce garlic capsules, to stimulate appetite, to lower high cholesterol and high blood pressure, to prevent arteriosclerosis, to kill children's parasites, as antiseptic and so on. Not all of these preparations are effective. If possible, raw garlic is the best remedy. Eating it every day will prevent colds and influenza, keep the blood vessels supple and healthy, keep the brain functioning and prevent dementia in old age. It will dissolve blood clots that sometimes form as a result of bruising. Garlic ointment will heal cracked nipples.

Dose

4 grams of fresh garlic or garlic capsules per day.

Contraindications

Some people suffer a burning sensation in the mouth and

intestine, nausea, sickness and odour from the breath and the body. Some people find it causes problems when applied to their skin. Garlic may interfere with some prescribed medicines.

Gentian Gentiana *asclepiadea*

Mythology

Gentian was sometimes called 'centaur's root' from watery Pelion, the land of the centaurs, where it grew luxuriantly in moist shady places. Several ancient writings, including those of Pliny the elder and Dioscorides mention the medicinal properties of gentian.

The name gentian comes from Gentius, the last King of Illyria, (near present-day Montenegro) from 181-168 BCE. Gentius, who was renowned for discovering the healing properties of gentian, was the first to suggest that it could be used against the plague. The second part of the binomial, asclepiadea refers to Asclepius. Ancient Greeks used Gentiana asclepiadea against poisonous bites, convulsions, liver and stomach complaints and internal bruising.

There are 400 different species of gentian, most of which grow in mountainous places. They are all protected and digging up the roots of the wild plants is strictly prohibited in the EU and Switzerland, where farmers have been growing gentian commercially for some time. Gentian grows slowly and can live up to 60 years because the bitter compounds in the entire plant, but much concentrated in their roots, keep them safe from grazing animals.

Botanical Description

Gentiana asclepiadea is a perennial plant that forms clumps of gracefully arching stems. It has lanceolate, willow-like smooth green leaves 5 cm long which spring from the upper leaf axils in pairs or threes. In late summer it produces trumpet-like deep blue flowers.

Healing Properties

Gentian root is bitter. When the tongue detects a bitter taste, it sends a message to the brain that something toxic needs to be eliminated fast. The brain then messages the salivary glands in the mouth to produce more saliva and the stomach to produce more digestive juices, in order to get rid of toxins more quickly. This reaction to bitter compounds stimulates the appetite and aids digestion. This is why traditional healers worldwide use the underground parts of various Gentiana species as remedies for poor appetite, digestive problems and to protect the liver.

In the mountainous regions of Europe people have been distilling a liquor with gentian and drinking it as an aperitif to stimulate the appetite and aid digestion, for hundreds of years. Liqueurs containing Gentian include Angostura bitters, Salers Aperitif, Aveze, Suze, Genzi, Genziana, Bittermens Amere Sauvage Gentian Liqueur, Cherry Rocher Gentiane and many more.

Chemical Constituents

Gentian contains flavonoids, flavonols and gallotannins. In 2011 Mihailovic found that the major compounds in the oil from the underground part of *Gentiana asclepiadea* were caryophyllene oxide, beta-damascenone and beta-ionone. The roots contain aldehydes, acids, aromatic compounds, esters, ketones, monoterpenes, diterpenes and sesquiterpenes. In 2013 Mihailovic and his team isolated the iridoids: sweroside, swertiamarin and gentiopicrine.

Research

Mihailovic in 2011 found that extracts of *Gentiana asclepiadea* were moderately anti-bacterial and anti-fungal but the essential oil from the root was more effective and the bacterium which was most susceptible to the root extracts was *S. aureus. S aureus* causes gastro-enteritis and poisoning and can be found in many different foods, according to Ahmadi in 2010. In 2003 Kumarasamy demonstrated that gentiopicroside, swertiamarin and sweroside were powerfully anti-bacterial.

In 2013 Mihailovic and his team found plenty of antioxidant compounds, such as flavonoids, flavonols and gallotannins, in Gentiana asclepiadea root, which were free radical scavenging and protected against lipid oxidation in vitro. They also protected cells from DNA damage in vitro.

Liver failure due to paracetamol overdose causes many deaths and life-threatening conditions every year, due to the fact that it is still an over-the-counter drug. In 2012 Suciu and her team demonstrated that Gentiana asclepiadea extract protected the liver of mice against paracetamol intoxication, probably due to the presence of erytro-centaurin. The extract was also anti-bacterial and anti-fungal. This does not mean that Gentiana asclepiadea extracts could save the lives of people who have overdosed on paracetamol, but it does indicate that gentian may protect the liver. In 2013 Mihailovitc found that gentian root extract protected the livers of rats. According to Chen in 2008 Gentiana scabra is used in Taiwan to treat chronic hepatitis. According to Zhao in 2010, many different species of gentian are used in Tibet to treat diseases of the liver and spleen.

According to Nayebi in 2016, another species of gentian, Gentiana olivieri is good at stimulating the appetite. According to Mirzaee in 2017, the root is anti-inflammatory, diuretic and protects the liver.

In 2016 Chen and his team analysed the clinical trials that had been carried out on patients suffering with vitiligo (a condition in which patches of skin have no pigment), using traditional herbal formulae, which contained gentian root, together with UV radiation. They found that the group taking the herbal formula improved more than the group which only had the UV treatment.

How to Use

Make a tea from the roots and rhizomes. Of course, you could always drink a gentian-based aperitif before dinner, if you have no objection to drinking a small amount of alcohol.

Dosage

1-4 g/day

Contraindications

Patients with ulcers or high blood pressure should not take gentian. Pregnant women should not use Gentiana, since it may cause them to miscarry. Do not exceed the recommended dose for this may cause headache, nausea, and vomiting.

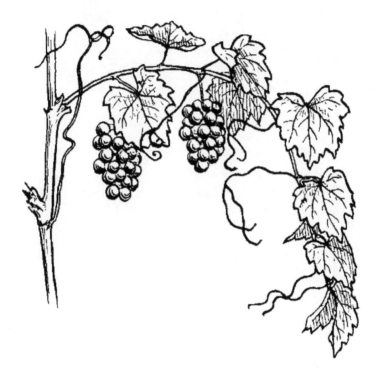

Grape vine *Vitis vinifera*

Mythology

The vine is inextricably linked with the god Dionysos, one of the most ancient Greek gods, whose name first occurred on a tablet from the Mycenaean period. Dionysos, who discovered the first grapevine, taught humans how to care for it and make wine, for he was the god of wine, grapes, ecstasy and sexuality. When his mother, Semele, was pregnant with him, Zeus's jealous wife, Hera persuaded Semele to prove her lover's divinity by asking him to appear in his real person. Zeus complied, but his power was too great for the mortal Semele, who was blasted with thunderbolts. Zeus saved his son by sewing him up in his thigh and keeping him there until he was ready to be born. Nonnus, in his Dionysiaca, writes that the name Dionysus means "Zeus-limp," a name chosen by Hermes for the new born baby, "because Zeus, while he carried his burden, lifted one foot with a limp from the weight of his thigh, and nysos in Syracusan language means limping." Hermes then took the baby to the maenads, who brought him up and became his female followers.

Dionysos represented the sap, juice, or lifeblood of nature and was surrounded by a retinue of satyrs and maenads. The satyrs were male nature spirits with little pointed horns, horse's ears and tails, and a permanent, exaggerated erection. The maenads were female nature spirits, who roamed the mountains and forests, performing frenzied, ecstatic dances as the god possessed them, before indulging in ritual feasts. When they were under the influence of Dionysos they could tear animals or people to pieces and possessed occult powers and the ability to charm snakes and suckle animals. Orfeus was one of their unfortunate victims.

Husbands watched, horrified, as their wives ran away to join the maenads and took to the hills, wearing fawn skins and crowns of ivy and shouting the ritual cry, "Euoi!" They formed holy bands and danced by torchlight to drum and pipe music, waving fennel wands bound with grapevines and tipped with ivy.

According to Nonnus, Dionysos's love, the Satyr Ampelos, rode on the back of a wild bull. He shouted excitedly to the full faced Moon:

"Give me best, Selene, horned driver of cattle! Now I am both - I have horns and I ride a bull!"

Selene looked with a jealous eye through the air, to see how Ampelos rode on the murderous marauding bull. She sent him cattle chasing gadfly; and the bull, pricked continually all over by the sharp sting, galloped away like a horse through pathless tracts. It threw the boy and gorged him to death.

The grieving Dionysus transformed Ampelos into a grape vine, evidently the highest accolade. According to Athenaeus the Hamadryad nymph of the wild grape vine was also called Ampelos. Dionysus also transformed one of his nurses, who was killed by the wicked Lykourgos, into a grape vine.

Botanical Description

The grapevine naturally climbs up anything it can cling onto, such as trees, its stems growing up to 35m in the wild, and spreading out branches. In the vineyard its growth is restricted through pruning. It grows slowly at first, as it forms an underground root system, but once it is established it grows fast. It forms a trunk with flaky bark and tendrils grow opposite leaves which are palmately lobed and hairy on the underside. Flowers form in dense panicles that develop into bunches of grapes. It is pollinated by wind, insects and self-pollination.

Healing Properties

Traditional healers in Europe use grapevine sap, juice, and

whole grape to treat pain, allergic reactions, inflammation, and to promote wound healing. Grape seed extract is produced by grinding up grape seeds and then either cold pressing them or steam distilling them. Cold pressing is always best, since it alters the healing compounds in the extract the least. Grape seed extract is antioxidant, anti-inflammatory, anti-bacterial, anti-fungal and protects the heart, intestines, liver and nerves.

People suffering from metabolic syndrome may have high blood pressure, diabetes, high levels of blood fats as well as cardiovascular diseases and stroke. Grape seed extract helps to prevent high blood fats, high blood sugar and high blood pressure, all risk factors involved in metabolic syndrome.

Acne-prone skin seems to be deficient in linoleic acid, so that sebum in the skin's pores becomes thick and sticky, which leads to blocked pores. Grape seed oil helps control acne by decreasing clogged pores. Since it is also astringent and antiseptic it will fight bacterial infections.

The antioxidants in grapeseed oil can help to prevent free radical damage to your skin caused by pollution and UV, and help protect your skin from skin cancer. Grapeseed oil contains polyphenols, which may help fight premature ageing.

Chemical constituents

Some of the most important compounds in grape seed extract are tannins, oligomeric procyanidins, catechins and epicatechins, as well as Vitamin E, and linoleic acid. Grape seeds contain high amounts of polyphenols, such as proanthocyanidins, which are potent antioxidants.

Grape seed and grape skin contain several active components including flavonoids, polyphenols, anthocyanins, proanthocyanidins, and the stilbene derivative resveratrol and trans-squalene. The flesh of the grapes contains several different sugars such as: glucose, fructose and galactose, as well as several different acids, such as: malic, tartaric, citric, isocitric, ascorbic.

Research

Resveratrol is a natural polyphenol in grape skins and also, to the delight of wine drinkers, in red wine. This compound has stirred up a great deal of excitement since it appears to have a number of healing properties. Several scientists have been investigating it, since it seems to be anti-carcinogenic, antioxidant, anti-diabetic, protects from atherosclerosis and perhaps most interesting of all, it may have anti-ageing properties. Most of the research leading to these conclusions was carried out on animals in the laboratory. For example, in 2007 Gruber found that it was antioxidant and when he fed it to nematode worms they lived longer. In 2012 Jun Park and team stated that resveratrol, had anti-aging properties and helped to prevent late onset diabetes. In 2006 Baur and team found that it protected rats from obesity and insulin resistance although they had been fed a high-calorie diet.

In 2011 Brasnyó and team carried out a small double-blind clinical trial with 19 patients suffering from type 2 diabetes. They gave resveratrol to half the patients and placebo to the other half. They found that the group who took the resveratrol had increased sensitivity to insulin.

Our cells have mitochondria in them, which generate energy. So, the more mitochondria we have, the more energy we can produce. According to Lagouge in 2006 resveratrol stimulates cells to produce more mitochondria and makes them more efficient. In 2010 Um and team found that it increased metabolic rate: the rate at which an animal uses energy. This is what we would expect as a result of more mitochondria producing more energy. So, the reason why Baur's rats did not gain weight was probably because the resveratrol increased their metabolic rate.

Resveratrol may help to improve memory and protect against

aging-related diseases such as Alzheimer's and Parkinson's, though no clinical trials have been carried out to see whether this is the case. I cannot help feeling that all this focus on a single compound is due to the fact that the pharmaceutical industry tends to produce single chemical medicines. These often have side effects, whereas plants produce a multitude of different compounds which act together, synergistically and are less likely to produce side effects.

Grape seed oil protects against radiation, according to Thorsten in 2008. In 2003 Jayaprakasha demonstrated that extracts of grape seeds inhibited bacteria and were antioxidant *in vitro*. In 2016 Akaberi and Hosseinzadeh demonstrated in the laboratory that polyphenols from grape seeds lowered high blood sugar, high blood fats and high blood pressure and protected the liver and heart. In 2010 Shivananda Nayak demonstrated that grape-skin powder speeded up wound-healing in rats. In 2011 Hemmati and team similarly demonstrated that grape seed extract promoted wound healing in rabbits. They suggested that the wound healing effect was due to the anti-inflammatory and antioxidant compounds in the extract. In 1999 Elsherbini patented a product containing trans-squalene, a grape seed compound, as an anti-viral compound for treating hepatitis C virus carriers.

Our bodies naturally produce the compound, nitric oxide. It is also emitted by vehicles, coal-powered power stations, burning oil, diesel, gas, and cigarettes. There is too much nitric oxide around and excessive amounts can be harmful to the cardiovascular system, the nervous system, the immune system and the skin, because it is extremely chemically reactive. *Vitis vinifera* contains compounds which stop our bodies producing nitric oxide, so in 2003 Cals-Grieson patented a series of anti-aging, sun tanning, after sun, and deodorant preparations containing *Vites vinifera* extract.

In 2016 Zeghad and team demonstrated that extracts of

freeze-dried grapes reduced pain in mice. In 2006 Naseri and team demonstrated that grape leaf extract had a relaxing effect on rat colon.

How to Use

It is much better to eat organic grapes whole, including the skin and pips, which both contain healing properties, than to drink grape juice. But do not eat excessive quantities of grapes, since they are loaded with sugar.

Take grape seed extract to improve your skin, to lower cholesterol and help to regulate blood pressure.

Use grape seed oil on your skin since it is lightweight and suitable for most skin types, including sensitive and acne-prone. Use it by itself, mix it into lotions or serums, or use it as a carrier oil. But do a spot test first to ensure you are not allergic to it. Use cold-pressed grape seed oil since it hasn't been heated, distilled, or chemically processed, all of which destroy some of its antioxidant, anti-inflammatory, and anti-microbial properties. Make sure that it is organic, so that it does not contain harmful pesticides and herbicides. It will help skin repair, speed the healing of wounds, reduce swelling after injury, and prevent muscle damage.

There are many cosmetic products on the market that contain grape seed oil, but you could make your own face creams and body lotions by simply buying a base cream and adding grape seed oil.

Dose

100-300 mg of grape seed extract per day.

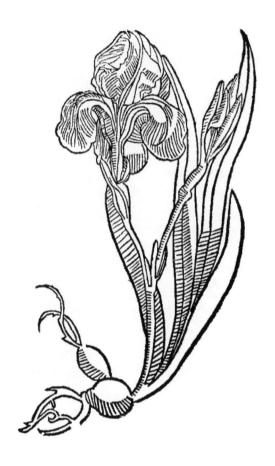

Iris, spp *Iris attica, I sintenisii, I orientalis, I germanica*

The common name iris originates from the Greek word for rainbow because irises flower in all the colours of the rainbow, according to Cumo in 2013. Iris, messenger of the gods, escorted the souls of mortals along the path made by the rainbow to the underworld.

The ancient Greeks scented their wine with perfumed iris rhizomes or extracted an aromatic oil for use in perfumes, ointments and salves. Pausanias described an ancient pharmaceutical laboratory in Boetia (Voiotia in modern Greece) where expert workers made pain-killing ointments from roses, lilies (Iris pseudacorus) and narcissi. One can imagine workers stoking marvellous distillation retorts with multiple orifices to collect the essential oils, while others mixed beeswax, almond oil and perfumed essential oils to make precious ointments, poured into tiny ceramic containers. Smoke and steam would have rendered the atmosphere almost impenetrable while tiny windows let oblique shafts of light penetrate the dark and dingy atmosphere.

Theophrastus and Dioscorides knew all about Orris Root (the root and rhizome of the iris, probably Iris germanica.) Dioscorides and Pliny say that the best came from Illyricum (the north western part of the Balkan peninsula.)

Botanical Description

There are about 300 species of iris. They either have bulbs or rhizomes (thick, creeping underground stems) and the flowers consist of 6 petal-like floral segments, the more erect inner ones called standards and the usually drooping outer ones called falls. They have sturdy swordlike leaves and their tall stems grow up to 90 cm with 3 to many flowers. There are also heavier, larger-flowered species in a full range of colours and combinations and dwarf bearded irises. Early flowering irises are a welcome sight in Greece after the winter months.

In Italy they grow fields of Iris germanica, Iris florentina and Iris pallida for the perfume industry. They dig up the rhizomes and when these are dried and peeled, they are known as orris root. When they are used for medicine the roots are known as rhizome iridis. When iris rhizomes are dried for less than two years and hydro-distilled this results in the production of resinoids, which smell like chocolate, or woody, leathery or hay-like, according to Roger in 2012. On the other hand, when iris rhizomes are dried for three years, the fats and oils in them degrade, releasing fragrant compounds called irones, which smell like violets. The essential oil from the three-year-old rhizomes, one of the most expensive, according to Basser in 2011, strengthens or enhances the fragrance of other aromatic herbs and prolongs their staying power.

Healing Properties

Traditional healers have used the roots and rhizomes of many *Iris* species to treat coughs, colds, bronchitis and as an anti-spasmodic. They use decoctions of the rhizomes to treat hormone-related diseases. The roots contain potent anti-cholinesterase, anti-cancer and anti-malarial compounds. Root decoctions loosen phlegm in the chest and lungs and act as expectorant, soothe sore throat and pacify coughing. Root decoctions also calm smooth muscle and control nausea, according to Rahman in 2003. Taken in small doses the root will relieve congestion and sluggishness in the liver.

It stimulates the gall bladder to secrete bile, and the mouth to secrete saliva, which in turn stimulates both the appetite, the stomach and digestive system and speeds up elimination through the bowel. It is also decongestant, expectorant, diuretic, carminative, purgative and emmenagogue. Eclectic herbalists used it as cathartic, alterative, vermifuge and diuretic. Ellingwood, in his American Materia Medica said iris root stimulated the glandular system, but cautioned not to exceed the dose, since high doses were toxic.

Chemical constituents

Scientists have isolated a multitude of compounds from Iris species but the main components are flavones, isoflavones, xanthones, quinones, terpenes and simple phenolics, with multiple biological activities. Iris extracts are rich sources of terpenoids, including iridal-type triterpenoids. *Iris germanica* also contains plant steroids such as beta-sitosterol and stigmasterol. Many of the compounds in *Iris species* are unique, such as the flavonoids, irigenin, irilone and iriflogenen which Lim isolated from Iris roots in 2016.

Research

In recent years there has been a considerable amount of research into the medicinal properties of Iris species, covering both flowers, leaves and rhizomes, most of it carried out in the laboratory. I will not try to cover all the research, which would take too long.

There are several stages in the development of cancer. Certain substances: pro-carcinogens, can be transformed into carcinogens by a human enzyme. In 2003 Wollenweber found that the Iris isoflavone compounds: irigenin, irilone and iriflogenen, prevented this enzyme from converting the pro-carcinogens into carcinogens, which indicates that iris root could protect us from cancer.

Some iris extracts, such as those from *Iris germanica*, are anti-inflammatory and antioxidant, according to Schutz in 2011, and contain anti-bacterial compounds, according to Orhan in 2003. In 2013 Huwaitat found that flower extracts of *Iris nigricans* were antioxidant. In 2016 Lim found that unique flavonoids from Iris were antioxidant, anti-mutagenic and anti-microbial. In 2011 Hacibekiroglu and Kolak found that extracts of fresh rhizomes and dried flowering aerial parts of *Iris albicans* were antioxidant and anti-cholinesterase. Extracts of *Iris suaveolens* were also antioxidant and anti-cholinesterase. Several scientists found that the roots were anti-bacterial and anti-fungal. In 2013 Ramtin demonstrated that the volatile oil from *Iris pseudacorus* was anti-bacterial.

In 2002 Wuttke patented a pharmaceutical composition containing tectorigenin, an isoflavone from *Iris germanica* rhizomes, for the treatment of hormone-related diseases. In 2001 Bonfils reported that iridals, triterpenoids isolated from *Iris germanica*, kill fish, tumour cells, snails and the bacterium that causes tuberculosis, as well as activating protein kinase C, which is involved in many different things, including immune responses, regulating cell growth and in learning and memory. In 2011 Basser reported that essential oil from Iris flowers was sedative, so he suggested that it could be used in aromatherapy. Also, in 2013 Mosihuzzman reported that *Iris loczyi* and *Iris unguicularis* contain compounds which inhibit a-glucosidase and might help manage diabetes and late diabetic complications.

This flurry of research into the medicinal properties of Iris spp has yielded interesting results. It might be interesting to carry out some clinical trials in order to ascertain how best to use Iris as a herbal medicine, but I have a feeling that the Pharmaceutical Industries will focus on the isolation of active compounds to develop as new pharmaceutical products.

How to Use
Make a decoction by boiling the powdered root 1-5 minutes in a cup of water or use a tincture of orris root, and take to loosen phlegm in the chest and lungs and to act as expectorant, sooth sore throat and pacify coughing. Take for its laxative effect on the bowels, to relieve congestion and sluggishness in the liver,

to stimulate the stomach and digestive system. Use together with other herbs to stimulate the lymphatic system and the kidneys to rid the body of toxins.

Use iris essential oil, diluted in a carrier oil in aromatherapy massage for its calming, relaxing effect.

Dosage

0.3-0.9g of powdered root.

Tincture of orris root: Take 6-12 drops in juice or water, 3 times a day.

Shake well. Store in cool dark place. Keep out of reach of children.

Contraindications

Pregnant and breast-feeding women should not take iris (orris) root. Some people are allergic to rhizome iridis though it seems to be safe for most people when taken by mouth, as long as you don't exceed the dose. There are no known side effects if the root is carefully peeled and dried. However, the fresh plant juice or root can cause severe irritation of the mouth, stomach pain, vomiting, bloody diarrhoea and severe skin irritation. There isn't enough information to know if the dried rhizome iridis might be safe when applied directly to the skin.

Mallow *Althaea officinalis*

The Greek name 'althaia' is derived from the words 'althos': a medicine, 'altho': to cure and 'althaiein': to heal. According to Mrs Grieve its family name Malvaceae is derived from the Greek malake, meaning soft. Dioscorides used the marshmallow for bruises, inflammations and to protect his patients from the bites of poisonous beasts.

Mythology

Althaea officinalis is named after Althaea, the daughter of King Thestius and Eurythemis. According to Hyginus, when her son Meleager was born, Clotho, one of the three fates, sang that he would be noble, Lachesis sang that he would be brave but Atropos, the third fate, looking at the brand burning on the hearth said:

"He will only live as long as this brand remains unconsumed."

When Althaea heard this, she leapt out of bed, put out the burning brand and buried it in the middle of the palace.

Meleager grew to be a well-respected prince. One spring Oeneus, Althaea's brother, sacrificed the first fruits of the seasons to all the gods, omitting Artemis by mistake. Furious Artemis sent a huge boar to ruin the land of Calydon. Meleager and the huntress, Atalanta, together with Althaea's brothers, rushed out of the palace, holding their spears aloft and hunted and killed the boar, so Meleager gave Atalanta the boar skin. Althaea's brothers snatched the skin from Atalanta and Meleager flew into a rage and killed both of his uncles. When Althaea learned what had happened, she went and dug up the brand and put it back on the fire, where it was consumed and Meleager died. Althaea then killed herself.

Botanical description

Althea officinalis has tall, stiff, velvety stems, up to 1.5 m high, with velvety leaves growing on alternate sides all the way up the stem. The leaves have 3-5 shallow lobes, folded like a fan. The flowers are pale pink with five broad petals and grow in clusters all the way up the stem from May to September. It is similar to hollyhock, the old-fashioned garden flower. For a botanical drawing of mallow please see my book: "The Healing Power of Celtic Plants."

Healing Properties

Everything about this plant is soft: its soft, velvety leaves and stem, its soft, soothing effect on the throat as it slips down, soothing the stomach and the rest of the digestive tract. Marshmallow is a demulcent, or soothing herb, because it contains large amounts of mucilage. According to Schultz in 1998, mucilage forms a protective layer on the lining of the throat and reduces the irritation of receptors, thus soothing a cough. Marshmallow is also expectorant, so particularly good for making a dry irritating cough productive. Demulcents, unlike opioid-based cough suppressants, are neither sedative nor addictive. It also soothes the digestive system, so has a calming effect on gastritis, gastric or peptic ulceration and enteritis, and specifically for gastric and duodenal ulcer. Marshmallow ointment soothes and softens grazes, cracks, inflammation and insect stings. It also soothes the urinary tract.

In 1989 the German Commission E approved both marshmallow leaf and root for irritation of the mouth and throat and dry cough. The Commission also approved the root for mild inflammation of the stomach lining.

For a list of the chemical constituents in the root, leaf and flower and for a description of the research that has been carried out on Mallow see my book: "Healing Plants of the Celtic Druids."

How to Use

Add marshmallow tincture to cough mixtures, for its wonderful soothing properties. It will calm the patient and make a dry cough productive. Take a warm infusion of the root, or tincture three times a day, to soothe a dry cough or take a spoonful of the syrup to allay an acute bout of coughing. Take an infusion to soothe colitis, acid indigestion and urinary stones. Rub marshmallow ointment on inflamed skin and joints, ulceration, stings and bites, neuralgia and inflamed breasts.

Contraindications

Marshmallow is safe in pregnancy and lactation. Do not take marshmallow for long periods of time since it could possibly reduce the absorption of other medicines.

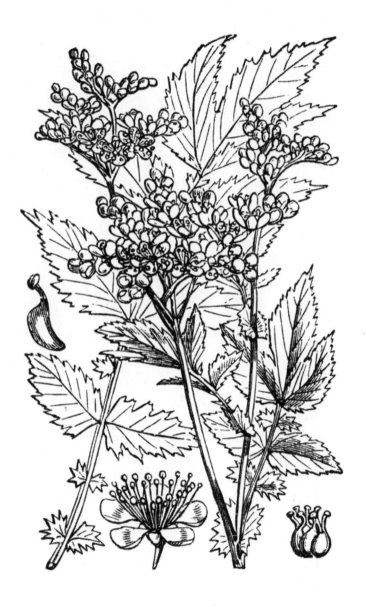

Meadowsweet *Filipendula ulmaria*

Theophrastus mentions meadowsweet, which grows in mountain pastures, was cultivated in the lowlands for use in festivals, celebrations and rituals. Pliny said:

"Meadowsweet comes after omphacium, which vines from the woods bear, and was spoken by us [before] in the discussion of unguents. It is most praised in Syria, from the white vine around the mountains of Antioch and Laodicea. It cools, is bitter, is poured on wounds, placed on the stomach, a diuretic, good for the liver, headaches, dysentery ... and for nausea: a drink with an obol's worth of vinegar. It dries up the flowing eruptions from the head, and it is most effective for defects, which are because of humidity [body composition, not weather]; for this reason, it is mixed with honey and saffron to address ulcers of the mouth and [to aid] the fundamental organs. It loosens the stomach, and heals the running of the eyes and maladies of the reproductive organs. Dissolved in wine it is good for the stomach; a drink from cold water it helps with the expelling of blood."

For a botanical description and a botanical drawing of meadowsweet please see my book: "Healing Plants of the Celtic Druids."

Healing Properties

Filipendula ulmaria's pain killing effect is due to salicylic acid, which is released from various compounds in the plant, such as salicyl-aldehyde and methyl-salicylate as they pass through the digestive system, according to Papp in 2008. Meadowsweet is diaphoretic, anti-inflammatory, astringent, antiseptic and analgesic. According to the American Gastroenterological Association (AGA), each year the side effects of non-steroidal anti-inflammatory drugs (NSAIDs) hospitalise over 100,000 people and kill 16,500 people in the U.S. alone. The most common side effects of aspirin include bleeding ulcers and tinnitus. Ironically, meadowsweet is commonly used by herbalists to heal the problems that aspirin creates. By isolating salicin from meadowsweet and willow and turning it into aspirin, the pharmaceutical industry has left out natural buffering agents found in the whole plant.

Unfortunately, few scientists have carried out any clinical trials with meadowsweet, so although we know that it contains many valuable compounds with painkilling, anti-bacterial and antioxidant properties, we do not have hard, scientific evidence that it is effective. However, herbalists have been using it to treat many painful conditions for centuries and swear that it works.

For a full list of the chemical constituents and a description of the research that has been carried out on meadowsweet see my book: "Healing Plants of the Celtic Druids."

How to Use

Take an infusion of the flowers to alleviate the pain of inflamed joints, for arthritis, rheumatism, headaches and neuralgia. The tannins and mucilage in it protect the wall of the gut, making it valuable for healing heartburn, gastritis, diarrhoea, enteritis, acid indigestion, peptic ulcers, and gastric ulceration. An infusion will help to relieve intestinal wind. Take meadowsweet infusion for colds, coughs and influenza. It relaxes the muscles and encourages sleep. Since it is gently diuretic it helps to rid the body of toxic wastes and uric acid so since it is also astringent and antiseptic, it helps clear up skin diseases.

Contraindications

Meadowsweet contains salicylates so it may increase the risk of bleeding when the patient is taking anti-coagulant or non-steroidal anti-inflammatory drugs (NSAIDs), or any anti-platelet medicines. Patients with salicylate or sulphite sensitivity should not use meadowsweet. Patients with asthma should use it with caution. Pregnant and lactating women should not take it.

Mistletoe *Viscum album*

Mistletoe figured prominently in Greek mythology and was used by heroes to access the underworld. Virgil describes Persephone opening the gates to the Underworld with mistletoe in her hand. The Trojan hero, Aeneas, took a piece of it with him when he visited the underworld to make sure that he would always be able to return to the world above. At the entrance to the underworld, he met the ghost of his father, who told him that Rome would one day dominate the Mediterranean. Protected by his mistletoe, he left the underworld and travelled to Italy, where he became the national hero of the Romans.

Pliny described how people believed that mistletoe would promote fertility and protect against poison. Theophrastus described mistletoe as an evergreen plant growing on pine and fir trees, spread by birds who eat the white berries. Marzell in 1923, suggests that combinations of aromatic plants and mistletoe were used to scent houses to protect them against lightening, spells and bad dreams. Dioscorides and Hippocrates used mistletoe to treat diseases of the spleen and menstrual problems. The goddess Athene used mistletoe to cure everything.

For a botanical description and a botanical drawing of mistletoe please see my book: "The Healing Power of Celtic Plants."

Healing Properties

The special compounds: lectins, viscotoxins and alkaloids, in mistletoe stimulate the immune system and inhibit cancer cells. For a full description of the chemical constituents of mistletoe and the research that has been carried out on mistletoe, please consult my book, "The Healing Power of Celtic Plants."

Peony *Peonia spp*

Mythology

The peony derives its name from an ancient Greek god of healing: Paeon, whose name is inscribed on a Linear B tablet at Knossos in Crete. Paeon, "the healing," is, according to Homer, the physician of the Olympian gods, who healed Hades and Ares with a healing balm on Mount Olympus after they had been wounded in battle at Troy.

"As quickly as white milk with rennet thickens
Likewise the blood in the wounds of Ares became, because of
Paeon's herbs."

After the time of Homer and Hesiod, the word Paeon became an epithet for Apollo and later Asclepius. Later still Paeon was applied to Apollo and Thanatos, or death, since they delivered men from the pains and sorrows of life, according to Sophocles.

According to another legend, Leto, the mother of Apollo, revealed to Paeon the virtues of a herb on Mount Olympus for easing childbirth, and this was called Peony.

Hekate, the healer, grew peonies in her magical garden in Colchis, on the shore of the Black Sea. It was a secret, hidden place, surrounded by high walls, where, with the help of her daughter, Medea, she cultivated magical poisonous plants, often mentioned by Homer.

Dioscorides described two kinds of peony, one called the male, with leaves like walnut (Juglans), and the other called the female with much more divided leaves like alexanders (Smyrnium), with different roots. The male roots being finger-like, while those of the female had swellings like an asphodel. In fact, what Dioscorides described as the male peony actually belongs to the Paeonia macula group, while the peony he called female belongs to the Paeonia officinalis group, i.e., two separate species. He prescribed 10-12 red seeds in wine to stop menstrual flow, but up to 15 in wine or mead to prevent nightmares, hysteria and pains of the womb. Pliny, who described it growing on shaded mountains, also mentioned its use against nightmares and Theophrastus, who also used peony, derided the idea that it should be dug up at night to avoid attack by a woodpecker. This was unfortunate since such stories were designed to terrify would be root gatherers and keep them away from this precious resource, thus preventing the eradication of the species.

Botanical Description

Peonies are unique, belonging to their own family, the Peonaceae. There are many different species of peony, several of which grow in Greece. All the Greek peonies die down completely for part of the year, with large buds on a subterranean root-stock from which fleshy roots descend into the earth. The roots may be tapering, as in P mascula, P clusii and P rhodia, or spindle shaped or rounded as in P officinalis, P parnassica and P peregrina, in which a slender string-like attachment growing from the rootstock becomes gradually or abruptly swollen, then narrows into a slender portion bearing the root hairs with the tubers hanging on strings or very thick threads as in Filipendula vulgaris.

At the base of the stem are several sheaths sometimes regarded as stipules but probably best compared to modified petioles. The flowering stem always has between 3 and 12 long-stalked alternate leaves without stipules. For example, P tenuifolia has usually 9-11 leaves, P mascula subsp russi usually 4-6. The leaves vary according to species but the basic type consists of a long petiole from which grow 3 primary petiolules, each with 3 primary segments or leaflets, so the whole leaf is divided into 9 segments. Some species have more complicated leaves with multiple divisions. In the Greek species the ultimate lobes have rounded or pointed tips and are smooth and hairless or very slightly hairy on the underside. The leaves are green in most species but red or reddish in P mascula subsp russi, P clusii and P rhodia. The stem usually grows to 25-35 cm in P. mascula and P clusii and to 60-80 cm in P peregrina.

The open flower may be bowl-shaped, at first almost round, as in P peregrina, to saucer-shaped with more widely spreading petals, as in P mascula subsp russi, and when fully open about 7-13 cm broad. P mascula subsp hellenica, P clusii and P rhodia always have white flowers, occasionally with a faint pink tinge towards the base. P mascula subsp russi and others have rose-pink or purplish flowers, but in P peregrina, the most spectacular of herbaceous peonies, they are a deep rich glossy red. P parnassica has very dark red flowers. Peony flowers have numerous stamens, either white or rose, with slender filaments and yellow anthers with very abundant yellow pollen. In the wild, large beetles crawl between the stamens and over the stigma eating the pollen. Peony flowers are particularly suited for beetle-pollination: they provide a broad landing area, have no complexity, often emit a somewhat fusty smell and offer their pollen lavishly. Since both beetles and peonies are of great antiquity, they have probably had a close association all through their history.

Healing Properties

People in China use peony root for gout, osteoarthritis, cough, cold, bronchitis and flu. Women use peony for menstrual cramps, polycystic ovary syndrome and PMS. It is also used to restore damaged liver, for upset stomach, to prevent hardening of the arteries, headache, nerve pain and chronic fatigue syndrome.

Chinese peony helps circulation, nourishes the blood, increases its production and helps to prevent thrombosis. It supports coronary blood-flow, reduces the amount of oxygen the heart needs to use and helps to prevent arrhythmia. Peony extract has aspirin-like effects and may prevent platelets sticking together. The Chinese herb, white peony (*Paeonia lactiflora*), reduces inflammation and balances the immune system, so providing help for rheumatoid arthritis. Peony (*Paeonia suffruticosa*) has been used in traditional Chinese remedies for dementia, Alzheimers and other neuronal diseases. It helps to regulate the menstrual cycle by rebalancing the female hormones. People in the Himalayas have been using the roots of the Himalayan Peony, *Paeonia emodi,* as a medicine for epilepsy traditionally for many centuries.

Chemical constituents

Peony species contain a cornucopia of healing compounds: monoterpenoid glycosides, flavonoids, tannins, stilbenes, triterpenoids and steroids, paeonols, and phenols. The roots of several *Peoni species* all contain unique compounds such as: paeoniflorin, benzoylpaeoniflorin, oxypaeoni-florin, paeonol, paeonoside, paeonolide, and apiopaeonoside. Peoniflorin is the major monoterpenoid glycoside. There are several different types of flavonoids: flavonols, anthocyanidins, chalcones, flavones, flavanone, and a flavan-3-ol. Peony seeds contain stilbenes. All parts of the plants contain triterpenes and steroids. The roots contain phenols.

Paeonol, the phytoestrogen paeoniflorin and the mixture of all glucosides of peony have already been established as new drugs.

Research

According to Lee in 2008, the Chinese herb, white peony, *Peoni lactiflora* is considered to be a new antioxidant source for treating neuronal diseases in China. In 2014 Yarnell found that *Paeonia lactiflora,* was a hormone modulator, was anti-spasmodic and reduced damage to the liver caused by the common rheumatoid arthritis drugs methotrexate and leflunomide.

In 2008 Nikolova demonstrated the anti-inflammatory effect of *Paeonia peregrina* flowers and root extracts *in vivo*. The extracts also helped the host to resist infection by the pneumonia bacterium. In 2013 Ding and team demonstrated *in vivo* that monoterpene glycosides and aromatic acids from *Paeonia suffruticosa and Paeonia lactiflora* stopped platelets sticking together, and inhibited inflammation and hemorrhage due to bacterial infection.

Several scientists have demonstrated that peony extracts are anti-fungal, anti-parasitic and anti-viral, including Abdel-Aty in 2007 and Au in 2001. In 2006 Tak demonstrated that the monoterpenoids in *Paeonia suffruticosa* root bark were more effective than Deet against the copra mite. In 2006 Lee demonstrated *in vitro* that *P Lactiflora* extracts were anti-viral against the Hepatitis B virus. Many scientists have demonstrated in the laboratory that peony extracts have a beneficial effect on the immune system, including Wang in 2007. Several people, including Liapina in 2000 and Hirai in 1983 have demonstrated that peony extracts protect the cardiovascular system.

Chinese traditional medicine uses peony to treat a wide range of symptoms, almost always in a combination of several other herbs. Many clinical trials have been carried out with herbal mixtures that included peony.

In 2008 Yuan and team found that a significant proportion of schizophrenic patients treated with a peony/liquorice mixture started to menstruate again, with less menstrual pain. Several of them stopped producing a milky discharge and acne also disappeared in some cases.

In 2012 Fang and his team in Taiwan carried out a massive survey of women with endometriosis, a very painful condition that occurs when the lining of the uterus starts to grow in other parts of the body. Thousands of women were included in the study which compared those who used traditional Chinese herbal medicine and those who did not. The herbs most often used in the herbal medicine included peony: Paeonia lactiflora. The herbs seemed to stop blood from clotting and to reduce build-up of tissue in the abdomen, reduce pelvic and abdominal pain, dark blood and clotting in menstruation. Unfortunately, there was no proof that the herbs stopped the endometrial tissues from migrating out of the uterus. In 2014 Arentz reviewed the use of herbal medicines to treat polycystic ovary syndrome, a complicated disease which can cause irregular menstruation and signs of excess male hormones, among other symptoms. He found that Tribulus and licorice, in combination with Chinese peony, and cassia caused the ovarian cysts and the male hormones to shrink while oestrogen increased in the patients who took these herbal remedies.

In 2009 Jang found that the symptoms of patients suffering from dysmenorrhoea: pelvic pain, lower back pain, painful breasts and headache during menstruation, improved after taking a traditional Korean herbal medicine composed of 12 herbs, including tree peony: Paeonia suffruticosa syn. P. moutan. In 2015 Yarnell also reported that a herbal remedy containing Chinese peony: Paeonia lactiflora, relieved the symptoms of dysmenorrhea.

In 2009 Xu found that white peony (*Paeonia lactiflora*) root and tree peony (*Paeonia suffruticosa*) were among the herbs used, together with conventional medicine, to increase survival rates and tumour remission rates in patients suffering from cervical cancer. In 2017 Ding reported that a Chinese herbal medicine containing four herbs, including Chinese peony *Paeonia lactiflora*, together with the chemotherapy drug camptothecin-11, decreased toxicity in normal tissue and helped to destroy cancer cells in liver and spleen tumours.

In 2011 Goto found that stroke victims who also suffered bleeding in their brains, heart attack, or paralysis for 12 months, who took a Chinese herbal medicine which contained peony: Peonia lactiflora and several other herbs remained more stable and deteriorated less than those in the control group. In 2016 Kim reported that the symptoms of patients with mild cognitive impairment (trouble remembering, learning new things, concentrating, or making decisions that affect their everyday life) improved after taking a herbal remedy containing 6 herbs, including Chinese peony Paeonia lactiflora. In 2006 Iwasaki and team found that a traditional herbal remedy containing eight different herbs, including tree peony: Paeonia suffruticosa, improved the cognitive score of patients with mild to severe dementia. At the end of the trial, they were better able to carry out daily activities and responded more quickly to care-givers.

In 2013 Fang and team found that infertile couples taking a herbal mixture containing ten herbs, including Chinese peony (Paeonia lactiflora syn. P. albiflora) root, produced more eggs and high-quality embryos compared with a control group.

In 2008 Salameh and team found that acupuncture and a herbal mixture including tree peony *Paeonia suffruticosa* improved the symptoms of 20 people with atopic dermatitis. In 2009 Tang reported that a Chinese herbal medicine containing peony root improved the symptoms of Hepatitis B. In 2013 Liu reported that a Chinese herbal remedy containing ten herbs, including Chinese peony: *Paeonia lactiflora*, reduced triglycerides in a group of patients with high triglyceride levels.

In 2015 Xu TCM reported that a Chinese herbal remedy containing twelve herbs, including white peony (*Paeonia lactiflora* syn. *P. albiflora*, Paeoniaceae) root, was non-toxic and improved fatigue in cancer survivors.

How to Use

You can add peony petals to salads or dry them and make them into teas. But I do not advise you to self-medicate with the roots because, although they are medicinal in minute quantities, they are also very toxic.

Rose gallic *Rosa gallica*

Flower of perfection, symbol of love, famed in many mythologies, highly prized by poets, the rose was dedicated to the Goddess of love and war: Ishtar in Babylonia, Isis in Egypt, Aphrodite in Greece and Venus in Rome. As Aphrodite emerged from the sea, roses grew from the foam. When she ran to save her lover, Adonis, from a wild boar sent by jealous Ares to kill him, she became entangled in thorn bushes and roses grew from her spilt blood. According to the Homeric Hymns, roses were among the flowers Persephone and her companion nymphs were gathering from a meadow when she was abducted by Hades.

Botanical Description

The gallic rose is a deciduous thorny shrub with bright pink flowers, which forms large patches. It was one of the earliest rose species to be domesticated by the ancient Greeks. It has slender, straight prickles, which occur in various sizes and frequency. The leaves are pinnately-compound, with three to seven bluish-green leaflets. The flowers are clustered one to four together, on glandular stalks. Wild plants usually have double corollas - two layers of petals.

Healing Properties

Rose petals lift the spirits with their perfume. They are mildly astringent and antioxidant, so can be used to strengthen a weak stomach and for diarrhoea, for sore mouth and throat. Rose hips are a valuable source of vitamin C in the winter. They are astringent, anti-bacterial, anti-inflammatory, antioxidant and used for colds, diabetes, diarrhoea, oedema, fever, gastritis, gout, rheumatism, sciatica. Rose hip powder, taken regularly will cure rheumatoid arthritis, prevent atheroschlerosis and lessen the pain of osteoarthritis.

For a full description of the chemical constituents and research that has been carried out on rose, see my book: "Healing Plants of the Celtic Druids."

Rosemary *Rosmarinus officinalis*

Mythology

The name rosemary comes from the Latin mare (sea) because rosemary grows by the sea, and rose from ros meaning dew, since it is often seen glittering with dew on the seashore. Aphrodite rose from the sea, where rosemary grew along the shore, surviving simply on the moisture in the air brought from the sea by gusts of wind. She generously gave rosemary to humankind.

Rosemary was associated with Mnemosyne, goddess of memory and the mother of the nine Muses, who presided over song. Minerva, the goddess of knowledge, is also associated with this herb. It was used at both weddings and funerals as it is today.

The ancients knew that rosemary strengthened the memory. Greek scholars wrapped rosemary round their heads while taking exams in order to enhance their memory and improve their performance.

For a botanical description and drawing of rosemary please see my book: "Healing Plants of the Celtic druids."

Healing Properties

Rosemary is diuretic, antiseptic, astringent and wound healing. It is antidepressant, tonic and calms the nerves. It is aromatic, helps to relieve flatulence, stimulates the liver and digestion and relaxes the smooth muscle of the intestines. Rosemary is rich in volatile oils, flavonoids and phenolic acids, which are antiseptic, anti-fungal and anti-inflammatory. It contains caffeic acid and its derivatives, such as rosmarinic acid, which are antioxidant. Rosmarinic acid in the extract of rosemary relaxes the smooth muscles of the trachea, the bronchi and the intestine and makes a dry cough productive. Rosemary inhibits some of the enzymes linked with memory loss. The German Commission E Monographs approve Rosmarinus officinalis rosemary for rheumatism, indigestion, loss of appetite and blood pressure problems.

Rosemary contains a number of aromatic compounds which inhibit acetylcholinesterase (AChE), the enzyme which breaks down acetyl choline (ACh). ACh is involved in sending and receiving messages in both the brain and the rest of the nervous system, therefore preventing the breakdown of ACh may delay the progression of Alzheimers disease.

In 1993 the US food and drug administration approved a drug called Cognex (tacrine) for treating Alzheimers. Tacrine inhibits AChE and clinical trials have demonstrated that about 25% of those taking it noticed some improvement. However, 25% of those taking it also suffered liver damage. In 2007 James Duke suggested that rosemary shampoo would be an excellent way to treat Alzheimers patients, since the anti-AChE compounds in rosemary would be absorbed through the scalp into the brain. Tacrine consists of one AChE inhibiting compound, whereas rosemary contains a dozen AChE inhibitors. In 1994 James Duke publicly bet his hair that rosemary shampoo would be as effective as tacrine as a treatment for Alzheimers.

For a list of chemical constituents and an explanation of the research that has been carried out on rosemary see my book: "Healing Plants of the Celtic Druids."

How to Use

Above all, use rosemary in food as often as you can. The great thing about rosemary is that you can pick it from a bush growing in your garden (if you have one) at any time of the year. But if you don't have a garden, supermarkets now sell fresh rosemary, which you can add to fish, meat or beans, or chop it up finely and add it to stuffings and sauces. Add rosemary to olive oil and leave to macerate for weeks. This will add a delightful flavour to your salad dressing. Roast vegetables are infinitely improved by the addition of rosemary. Add rosemary to soups. If you bake bread try adding sun-dried tomatoes, finely chopped rosemary and chopped onions to your dough for a Mediterranean flavoured bread.

Use an infusion for colds, coughs, influenza, indigestion, rheumatic pain, headaches, colic, depression and as an anti-spasmodic in renal colic and menstrual pain. Use it to relieve flatulence, stomach cramps, constipation and bloating. Use it to stimulate the liver and gall bladder. It will help to regulate the release of bile which will aid digestion and improve the absorption of nutrients from food. Use as a mouth wash to sweeten your breath, remove bacteria and prevent gingivitis.

Dilute the essential oil in a carrier oil to massage aching joints. Use on the skin as an antiseptic and to heal wounds, to cure eczema, dermatitis, oily skin and acne. Add rosemary essential oil to face creams and moisturisers to tone your skin. Rosemary oil and rosemary infusion help to stimulate hair follicles, if you use them regularly, making hair grow longer and stronger and slowing down premature hair loss. Rosemary massage oil, made with olive oil, nourishes the scalp and removes dandruff. Use rosemary essential oil vapour to lift your spirits, stimulate your brain, calm your nerves and improve concentration. It is a good remedy for depression, mental fatigue and forgetfulness. Add essential oil of rosemary to your shampoo to invigorate your brain and brighten your thoughts and feelings. Use relaxing, calming rosemary aromatherapy to de-stress.

Contraindications

Fresh rosemary leaves in food and as an infusion are quite safe. The essential oil of rosemary is potent and should not be taken internally in large doses since it may cause gastrointestinal and kidney disturbances. Essential oil of rosemary can irritate the skin, if it hasn't been adequately diluted with a carrier oil. You should not take phenolic-rich extracts of rosemary long term because they reduce the uptake of dietary iron. Pregnant and breastfeeding women should not use it.

St John's wort *Hypericum species*

Mythology

According to Dioscorides Chiron the centaur was particularly fond of St John's wort, which grew wild on Mount Pelion, where he lived in his cave. He used it on wounds.

For a botanical description and botanical drawing of St John's wort please see my book: "The Healing Power of Celtic Plants."

Healing properties

St John's wort can be used for mild depression and is safer than any of the pharmaceutical anti-depressants. It is especially good for the symptoms of menopause. Both the oil and the ointment are antiseptic and anti-inflammatory and astringent.

For a full description of the chemical constituents and research that has been carried out on St John's wort, see my book: "The Healing Power of Celtic Plants."

How to Use

Take the tincture or pills as an anti-depressant, to give you more energy and enthusiasm.

Use the tincture together with other soothing herbs, such as mallow, for inflammation of the internal organs. It will help relieve irritable bowel syndrome, aid the digestion and disinfect the gut.

Make a hypericum oil by covering the flowers with oil in a jar and leaving in the sunlight until it turns red. The addition of wax with turn the oil into an ointment. Use the oil or ointment to heal wounds, sores, ulcers, burns and swellings. It will speed up the healing process.

Valerian *Valeriana dioscoridis*

Dioscorides used valerian as a sedative and anti-epileptic, although he thought it smelt disgusting (and it does). There are approximately 250 species of valerian and most of them are used as herbal medicines. For a botanical description and botanical drawing of valerian please see my book: "The Healing Power of Celtic Plants."

In 1988 Houghton reviewed the chemical constituents of the different species and came to the conclusion that they all contained valepotriates, which have a sedative effect. Valerian is used to lower blood pressure and heart rate, to regulate the heart beat and prevent arrhythmia, to regulate lipid levels in the blood, as an anti-depressive and as an anti-anxiety herb.

For a description of the main Chemical Constituents and research that has been carried out on valerian, see my book: "The Healing Power of Celtic Plants."

Violet sweet *Viola odorata*

Mythology

Pindar, in his Olympian VI describes the birth of Iamos, son of Apollo and the nymph Euadne and his subsequent abandonment. His mother left him lying in the Arkadian wilds on a bed of violets, where serpents fed him honey. Eventually he was discovered by passing shepherds who named him Iamos after the violet (ion) bed.

People have been presenting bouquets of violets to the beloved throughout the ages and the ancient Greeks, who considered that violets were a symbol of fertility and love, made them into love potions. Gerard tells the tale of the 'young demosell, Io, that sweete girle, whom Jupiter courted' then 'he had got her with child.' After she had given birth, he turned her into a 'trim heiffer,' according to Dodoens, to protect her from the jealous eyes of Hera. He made violets grow as fragrant food for her. (Small consolation after being raped and turned into a cow!)

In the version of the story in which Zeus transformed Io, the deception failed, and Hera begged Zeus to give her the heifer as a present, which, having no reason to refuse, he did. Hera then sent Argus Panoptes, a giant who had 100 eyes, to watch Io and prevent Zeus from visiting her. So, Zeus sent Hermes to distract Argus. According to Ovid, Hermes lulled him to sleep with his panpipes, then, when Argus was safely sleeping, Hermes killed him. Zeus freed the unfortunate Io, who was still a cow.

Since love is associated with the heart and the spurned lover is 'broken hearted,' the ancient Greeks gave violet infusions as a tonic for the heart.

Botanical Description

It is a small, perennial plant with a stout rootstock, found in hedgerows, rough land and margins of woodlands. The leaves grow on stalks in a rosette from the root and are heart shaped and hairy with an oval stipule. The flowers are dark purple or white, have five petals and hang down from a curved stalk. The lowest petal has a prominent nectar-filled spur and the five sepals have basal appendages. It sends out long, creeping stolons, from which fresh plants grow. It has a beautiful, delicate scent.

Healing Properties

Violet flowers, leaves and roots store a cornucopia of valuable compounds with all sorts of healing properties. The mucilage in violet is soothing and anti-inflammatory, the saponins in the roots are expectorant, the salicylic acid eases pain and brings down a fever and the whole plant is anti-bacterial. The quercetin and scopoletin in the plant are anti-asthmatic. The rutin in the flowers helps maintain and strengthen the walls of the capillaries, so can help treat varicose veins. Viola odorata is diaphoretic, diuretic, laxative, emollient, antipyretic, sedative, anti-bacterial, antioxidant, protects the liver and lowers cholesterol.

For a full description of the chemical properties and research that has been carried out on violet, see my book: "The Healing Power of Celtic Plants."

Part 4

Poisonous Plants
in Greek Myth

Many of the most fascinating plants used by the ancient Greeks are highly poisonous. In antiquity, people used naturally occurring toxins to wage primitive and relatively sophisticated forms of chemical and biological warfare. As far back as the time of the Hittites of Asia Minor warring armies used toxins to gain an advantage over their enemies. The ancient Greeks used a wide variety of poisonous plants, venomous insects and reptiles, pathogens and toxic chemicals.

Ancient healers also used toxic plants as medicine, carefully administering small doses to heal many symptoms. Surgeons who practiced in the Asclepeion almost certainly administered narcotics such as opium and mandrake to patients in the dormitories to induce sleep thus enabling them to perform surgery unhindered by the screams of their patients. Ancient peoples were extremely aware of the powerful effects of plants. They were in awe of those who had plant knowledge, in many cases afraid. Anyone could go to a wise woman, witch or healer and ask for a lethal potion to slip into an enemy's dinner or drink.

Many of the poisonous plants had psychoactive properties and were used as hallucinogens. These substances were called *entheogen*, from the Greek *en* (full of), *theo* (god), and *gen* (create). Initiates in the Eleusinian Mysteries took *kykeon*, a psychoactive secret potion that induced visions and the state of ecstasy and divine communication. Participants who experienced marvellous visions were known as *epoptai*, or beholders. Famous figures including Plato, Aristotle, Pausanias, Sophocles, and Pindarus participated in the Eleusinian Mysteries.

Aconite, whose genus name *Aconitum*, derives from the Greek *akoniton* (without earth) grows on rocky ground. They also called it *lykoktonon* (wolf-slaying) because they coated their arrows with aconite when they hunted wolves. Its leaves and roots are extremely toxic and were used by the ancients as a poison since it contains the alkaloid, aconitine, which paralyses muscles and nerves.

According to Ovid, one of Hercules' twelve labours was to fetch Cerberus, the gigantic three-headed hound of Hades, with a mane of snakes and a dragon's tail, who guarded the entrance to the underworld. When Hercules found Cerberus, he grabbed him by the throat and wrestled him to the ground, then picked him up and threw him over his shoulders and took him back to King Eurystheus. As he walked, carrying the hound, a stream of spittle hung from Cerberus's mouth, which, when it touched the ground, caused the first aconite plant to grow. Again, according to Ovid, Medea attempted to poison Theseus with aconite dissolved in wine.

The name *Bryonia* derives from the Greek *bryo*, meaning shoot, possibly because it grows so fast.

The fertile flowers of black bryony (*Tamus communis*) produce shiny, red berries which are very attractive to small children, and toxic. I think I may have eaten some when I was a child which resulted in my mother making me drink a strong salt solution in order to make me vomit. Not a pleasant experience!

Dioscorides prescribed the red berries for freckles and skin blemishes and called it the '*ampelos agria*' (wild vine). He said that some people called white Bryony (*Bryonia dioica*) '*ophiostaphulon*' (snake's grape-cluster) referring to its toxicity. However, he also said that the root, leaves and fruit could be used as medicine, for external ulcers and abscesses, skin injuries, epilepsy, snake-bite and so on, but warned that only very small doses could be used. Exceeding the prescribed dose would cause madness. Hippocrates used bryony root for tetanus. Who knows whether it would have worked?

The ancient Greeks cultivated the castor oil plant: (*Ricinus communis,*) *kastorelaio* in Greek. Dioscorides called it *Kroton* (tick) because its seeds looked like a dog's tick (*ricinus* in Latin). He described the process of extracting oil from the seeds and said that it was not fit for food but could be used externally in medicine. He said castor oil was a drastic purgative and good for use as a lighting fuel. The seeds, which contain three toxic proteins ricin A, B and C, are highly poisonous and three large seeds are enough to kill an adult man.

Dioscorides described the toxic properties of deadly nightshade (*Atropa belladonna*):

> *"drinking one dram (3.5 ml) of the juice in wine results in pleasant hallucinations which can, if 2 drams (7 ml) are drunk, last as long as 4 days. 4 drams (14 ml), equivalent to 10 or 12 berries are lethal. Children will die from eating far fewer berries."*

The name of the genus, *Atropa,* is derived from the goddess Atropos, one of the three Moirai, goddesses who decided the fate of every human. Clotho spun the thread of life; Lachesis measured its length and Atropos held the shears with which she cut it and it was she who decided how each human would die. *Belladonna* is Italian for beautiful lady, because Italian ladies used to drop the juice from the berries into their eyes to dilate their pupils. Atropine, an active compound from belladonna, is still used today to dilate the pupils of patients.

Giant fennel (*Ferula communis*) is sacred to Prometheus, who, according to Hesiod, tricked Zeus into accepting the bones and fat of a sacrifice instead of the meat. So, Zeus hid fire from mortals. Prometheus took a fennel stalk and secretly stole fire from the forge of Hephaestus. Since the pith inside the stem of the fennel stalk smoulders very slowly without burning the outside of the stalk, he was able to bring fire to earth inside the fennel stalk. When Zeus found out he chained Prometheus to the summit of the Caucasus to punish him. An eagle devoured his liver each day and each day it renewed itself. Poor Prometheus was immortal so he had to suffer eternally, but he was saved by Chiron the centaur, who renounced his immortality in order to end his own suffering from his incurable wound.

Fennel-stalk torches were used in the Promethean torch-race festival. The *thyrsus* carried by his attendants and participants in the ceremonies associated with his worship was a long fennel stalk, often entwined with ivy and topped by a conifer cone. The god had ordered his followers to only use the stems of fennel, so that they would not hurt each other during their drunken quarrels.

Giant fennel was also dedicated to Dionysos.

According to the Pharmacy historian Julius Berendes in 1891, hellebore (*Helleborus species*) is the most famous drug in the Greek *Materia Medica* because of its many healing properties. The ancients distinguished two kinds of hellebore: the white and the black. Pausanias mentions an episode of biological warfare in the 6th century BCE when Solon of Athens poisoned the water supply with hellebore, during the siege of Krissa.

According to Apollodorus, Proetus's daughters were driven mad because they would not accept the new rites of Dionysus. They believed that they were cows and wandered the land, mooing. Finally, the seer Melampus cured them with hellebore. Alternatively, Melampus, who wanted to stop women from practicing the cult of Dionysus, obtained some milk from a goat that had eaten hellebore and fed it to them. I cannot believe that a goat, a highly intelligent animal, would eat hellebore. Nor can I believe that the followers of Dionysus would drink such evil tasting milk! But then again it is a myth. The toxicity of hellebores is mentioned in the Hippocratic writings:

"Convulsions following the administration of hellebore are fatal."

Hellebores kill, but before doing so they have a few side effects, including nausea and diarrhoea, and since Greek physicians believed in purging their patients, they would use hellebore for this purpose. It was a tricky business giving a small enough dose to purge the patient since a fraction too much resulted in convulsions and death. Despite this one of the most famous prescriptions in the Hippocratic writings is for hellebore to treat a mental disease called phrenites (possibly a form of schizophrenia), which most commonly strikes in the spring, and makes the patient feel afraid, see terrible things and have frightful dreams. They used hellebore as part of a drink to clean out the patient's head (and presumably his stomach).

Hemlock (*Conium maculatum*) gains its genus name: *Conium* from the Greek word *Konas*, meaning to whirl about, because the plant, when eaten, causes vertigo and death. The species name, *maculatum*, is Latin for spotted, and refers to the stem-markings.

Plato famously described the poisoning of Socrates with hemlock, when he was condemned to death by the law of Athens. Pliny added caustically that hemlock had a salutary effect on many people. He said:

"Hemlock, too, is a poisonous plant, rendered odious by the use made of it by the Athenian people, as an instrument of capital punishment: still, however, as it is employed for many useful purposes, it must not be omitted. ... The seed is crushed, and the juice extracted from it is left to thicken in the sun, and then divided into lozenges. This preparation proves fatal by coagulating the blood—another deadly property which belongs to it; and hence it is that the bodies of those who have been poisoned by it are covered with spots. It is sometimes used in combination with water as a medium for diluting certain medicaments. An emollient poultice is also prepared from this juice, for the purpose of cooling the stomach; but the principal use made of it is as a topical application, to check defluxions of the eyes in summer, and to allay pains in those organs. It is employed also as an ingredient in eye salves, and is used for arresting fluxes in other parts of the body: the leaves, too, have a soothing effect upon all kinds of pains and tumours, and upon defluxions of the eyes."

Hemlock has a disagreeable mousy smell, especially when it is bruised. The whole plant is poisonous. People have mistakenly eaten the leaves for parsley, the roots for parsnips and the seeds for anise seeds with fatal results. Hemlock contains eight piperidine alkaloids, including the highly toxic g-coniceine and coniine.

Henbane *(Hyoscyamus niger)*, derived from the Greek words *hyos* and *cyamos*, signifying hog's bean, since hogs apparently can eat it with impunity, is mentioned in the Ebers papyrus. It was also used by Assyrian and Babylonian priests as a powerful hallucinogen. In Greece, treatises written by Xenophon and Dioscordes refer to its intoxicating properties. According to Robert Graves', The Ancient Myths of Greece in 1955, it was believed that some souls of the dead roamed the banks of the river Styx at the entrance to Hades. These wraith-like spirits wore garlands of henbane to warn the living of the dangers of this plant. Apparently, Hercules discovered the hallucinogenic properties of white henbane. Dioscorides used the seed and leaves pounded and soaked with hot water to deaden pain and procure sleep. He preferred the white henbane to other species of henbane which he said could cause madness. Celsus and others, who lived in the same period, used it for the same purpose, internally and externally, though Pliny declared it to be:

"Of the nature of wine and therefore offensive to the understanding."

According to Mrs Grieves in 1931, an old writer says:

"If it be used either in sallet or in pottage, then doth it bring frenzie, and whoso useth more than four leaves shall be in danger to sleepe without waking."

Hyoscyamus contains tropane alkaloids, plant toxins that

are naturally produced in several plant families including Solanaceae (e.g., mandrake, henbane, deadly nightshade, Jimson weed.)

Datura (*Datura stramonium*) and belladonna (*Atropa belladonna*) were both used in Mesopotamia and Classical Greece.

Theophrastus and Aristotle mention the narcotic effects of *Mandragora officinalis*. In ancient Egypt there are paleo-ethnobotanical and artistic images of mandrake, as well as written papyri, which show that it was used ritually. The scenes depicted seem to represent ritual healing, in which a priest guides the souls of the living and the dead. These plants are represented in secret books of ritual magic, along with opium poppy, as 'vehicles to ecstasy.' There always was a relationship between altered mental states and communication with the gods and between healing and magic. According to Boguet in 1971, from very early times, the mandrake root was associated with a human form. The origin of the word *Mandragora* or mandrake is related to the Indo-European and Persian for man, *giyā* meaning "man plant," according to the Oxford English Dictionary. Mandrake's physiological effects on humans caused it to become a legend. Cuneiform tablets in the library of the palace at Nineveh show that it was used in Assyria, and a bas-relief from the reign of Amenhotep III shows that it was used as an anaesthetic in Egypt.

In ancient Egypt they used to brew mandrake beer to use as medicine and magic. According to R. Campbell Thompson, Egypt's chief deity, Ra, sent the goddess Hathor to slay all people, which she began to do. He began to regret his order and asked Hathor to stop but she replied:

"By thy life when I slaughter men then is my heart right joyful!"

So, Ra sent to Elephantine for a large supply of mandrake, asked a miller to brew beer and mix it with crushed mandrake and human blood from the dead. While Hathor slept, Ra ordered a courier to carry 7,000 jars of mandrake beer and to empty them to cover the ground four-hands deep. Awakening to resume her carnage, Hathor drank the beer tasting of human blood and mellowed. She fell into a drunken stupor and when she woke up, she relaxed and stopped killing humans. Ra ordered that from that day on, on Hathor's feast day, everyone should drink mandrake beer and then sleep.

In ancient times Mandrake was considered an invaluable aid in reversing infertility. But it was also associated with the Devil or Evil, going back to the male devil god, Namtar.

Hannibal the Carthaginian general (247–182 BCE) constantly at war with Rome, retreated from one particular battle, leaving behind a feast with wine drugged with mandrake. The enemy drank, slept, and was ambushed when Hannibal's troops returned, according to Stewart in 2009.

Columella and Pliny say that mandrake is also called *"circaeon,"* after Circe, goddess of love, who was originally associated with Isthar, the Assyrian Inanna counterpart. Dioscorides also gave mandrake's synonym as *Circaia*, "the Circe plant," possibly because she used a magic potion containing mandrake to transform Odysseus's crew into pigs, according to Homer.

Theophrastus described how drug dealers and root gatherers (*pharmakopōlai* and *rhizotomoi*) drew three circles around the mandrake with a sword, and cut it when they faced westward, dancing around the plant chanting as "many things as possible about the mysteries of love." Then they tied a dog to the mandrake, threw a piece of meat out of the dog's reach so that it would run to get it and pull the mandrake up, while the root gatherer covered his ears. The dog would die from the sound of the shrieking mandrake. This is yet another example of a scare story to stop would be root gatherers from depleting an already rare source of a valuable herb. In Dioscorides's Juliana Anicia there is an image of Dioscorides, seated, pointing to a mandrake held by Epinoia, the personification of Thinking, while in the foreground is a dog.

Dioscorides instructed that mandrake juice should be mixed with sweet wine and three *cyathoi* (approx. 0.137 litres) for those about to undergo surgery:

"For they become unaware of the pain because they sink into deep sleep."

The tropane alkaloids in it stopped the enzyme cholinesterase from breaking down acetylcholine, which caused the smooth muscles relax. He probably administered the potion drop by drop, slowly, observing the patient closely until they began to slip into unconsciousness. It was a highly skilled business, giving the patient enough to send them to sleep, but being careful not to overdose, since the results would have been fatal.

The Greek society of Anaesthetists uses the mandrake as its emblem.

Mandrake contains more than eighty compounds, including the deadly atropine, hyoscyamine and scopolamine. Very small doses induce a coma. Any more results in death.

Hippocratic Works state that mandrake was a strong narcotic and sedative. Pliny the Elder (23–79 CE) wrote that it should be "given before operations to dull the sense." It was prescribed for quartan fever (malaria) mixed with wine and drunk after the 4th day when the patient needed to rest, according to Hobbs. It was also prescribed for madness with a tendency to suicide, according to Dioscorides, for vaginal bleeding, to help the woman to sleep, according to Soranus, as a plaster for an inflamed rectum, according to Dioscorides, for convulsions, according to Riddle.

Theophrastus includes *Datura* in a list of four plants that induce sleep (*hypnos*) and act as a love potion (*philtron*) and provides the following information:

> *"Of this three twentieths of an ounce in weight is given, if he is to go mad outright and have delusions; thrice the dose if he is to be permanently insane...four times the dose is given, if the man is to be killed."*

The oracle at Delphi used the vapours of hallucinatory plants in order to enter into a trance. She would prepare by sitting by a crack in the rock from which intoxicating vapours arose, chewing bay leaves, or opium and datura, inhaling smoke from a variety of plants, and drinking water from a specific source, after which she would prophesy in an ecstatic trance state.

Some people say that Narcissus (Narcissus poeticus) derives from the Greek word narke, meaning to benumb, for the narcotic properties of its bulb, the most toxic part of the plant. It contains lycorine, an alkaloid known for its ability to induce vomiting and gastrointestinal cramping.

Ovid tells the story of Narcissus in his Metamorphoses. Even as a baby Narcissus was loveable but he grew up to become the most beautiful young man, poised on the edge of manhood, attractive to both men and women. But because of his pride he rejected the love of everyone. The nymph Echo saw him running through the forest, hunting, and fell in love with him but she could only repeat what he said. Narcissus, followed by Echo, found himself in a cool, grassy place with a beautiful pool with a perfectly still surface. He was thirsty and bent down to drink. As he raised himself up, the surface cleared and he saw himself for the first time reflected in the water. He was so entranced that he remained suspended in time, staring at his reflection, completely and utterly in love with it. He attempted to kiss and embrace his reflection, but he could not. Echo pitied him, echoing his cries. Gradually he wasted away, frustrated with desire and died. His body was transformed into a Narcissus poeticus, a flower which bends over, as though admiring its own reflection.

Homer describes how Zeus asked Gaia to grow the narcissus in order to temp Kore, who was with her companion nymphs gathering flowers in a springtime meadow. As she picked the narcissus a great gaping hole appeared in the earth, out of which erupted Hades, who grabbed Kore and carried her down to the underworld. The narcissus, necessary agent for greater self-awareness propelled Kore on a path of self-knowledge, autonomy and empowerment. She was transformed from a young innocent into Persephone, queen of the underworld. Eventually she returned to the upper world for part of each year and subsequently travels between the two realms, and through Demeter's inauguration of the Mysteries, she provides humans with recurring access to the underworld. The seductive power of the narcissus made these connections and transformations possible.

The opium poppy, whose Latin binomial, Papaver somniferum, means the "sleep-bringing poppy," is the king of medicinal plants, containing a veritable cornucopia of active compounds, which can be used by health professionals for a multitude of medical needs. The World Health Organisation lists medicines derived from the opium poppy as essential drugs, because they provide the most effective pain relief. Statues of Cretan-Mycenaean goddesses with poppy capsules demonstrate that people recognised the healing properties of poppies in ancient times, when goddess worship was still the order of the day. When Persephone was taken off by Hades, Demeter soothed her grief with the narcotic juice of the opium poppy.

The followers of Hippocrates used the capsule as well as the juice of several kinds of poppy. Dioscorides provided detailed instructions on making opium, as well as how to detect adulterations and imitations of the drug. He pounded the poppy heads with the leaves, pressed them, crushed them in a mortar with pestle and made pills out of the resultant paste. According to him a pill the size of a small pea would relieve suffering, bring sleep and comfort in the case of long illnesses but excessive consumption would eventually kill the patient.

Helen of Troy gave a pain-soothing drink, probably containing opium, called 'nepenthes' to Telemachus and his companions to help them to forget their dead companions. Poppy flowers adorned the revellers at festivals in honour of Demeter and poppy seed cakes featured in the mysteries, which may also have used opiates. Hypnos, the god of sleep, dripped poppy juice from his wand. Demeter loved a youth called Mekon. When he died, she transformed him into a poppy flower.

The opium poppy may have done as much damage to humanity as good, due to its addictive properties. For a full description of the Opium Wars in China, see my book: "Healing Plants of the Celtic Druids."

The yew tree (Taxus baccata) was sacred to the Erinyes, three goddesses of retribution and vengeance, predating the time of Zeus and the other Olympians. Who knows how they were depicted in ancient, pre-mythological times, but by the time the Helenes had imposed their gods on the ancient religion, the Erinyes had been transformed into monstrous crones, sinister women dressed in black with large wings, and bodies around which poisonous snakes circled. Their job was to punish men who committed heinous crimes. When Cronus castrated his father Uranus, the Erinyes were born from the drops of blood that fell onto Gaia, the earth. They could inflict madness upon any person who killed their own father or mother. The only way to placate the wrath of the Erinyes was to atone for the crime and engage in ritual purification. A victim seeking justice could call down the curse of the Erinys upon the criminal. They used a yew branch to drip purifying drops of water and as a flaming torch.

The yew tree was also sacred to Hekate, whose sacred tree of death roots in the mouths of the dead to release their souls, and absorbs the odours of death itself.

In Macbeth, Shakespeare referred to the contents of Hekate's cauldron as "slips of yew, silver'd in the moon's eclipse..." In Hamlet Shakespeare speaks of "hebenon, the double-fatal yew'" poison which Hamlet's uncle pours into the king's ear.

Paclitaxel, a compound isolated from Yew bark, is a major anti-cancer drug

Conclusions

When I began to research this book, I was not at all surprised to discover a host of sacred trees, for I knew that in prehistoric times tree worship was common to the whole of Europe, if not most of the world. But I was surprised by how many of these trees had well-known medicinal properties. The flowering plants and shrubs used by the ancient Greeks as medicine are even more numerous than the trees, so I have chosen just a few for this book.

Small groups of people in antiquity chose to settle in this beautiful place, living in harmony with their environment, eating the fruits of the trees that grew luxuriantly around them, hunting the animals that roamed in the woods and fishing in the rivers and sea. These early tribal people paid attention to the spirits of trees, rivers, mountains and animals and passed down by word-of-mouth myths about their goddesses and the world they lived in. Over time the myths began to be recorded and the goddess religion was overrun by a patriarchal religion with fierce gods.

The first healers were probably women who used herbs, ritual and incantations. Then by the time myths began to be recorded, mythical physicians such as Chiron, the wounded centaur, began to appear. He taught the great Asclepius, whose worship led to the creation of Asclepeia, where the sick came to be healed through dreaming with snakes. At around this time the first recognisable physicians began to practice, both within the Asclepeia and elsewhere, sometimes using surgery on the sleeping patients. People had always used herbs and these early surgeons knew how to induce a dreaming state with the use of narcotic plants, such as the opium poppy and mandrake. Over the next few hundred years herbal medicine, together with the names and descriptions of the healing plants, began to be recorded, as well as the methods of healing.

Ancient Greece, with its rich diversity of ecosystems and plants, was the birthplace of Western medicine and botany, the first botanists listing the medicinal plants together with botanical drawings. But whereas western medicine today focusses on drug-based cures and surgery to treat diseases, ancient Greek physicians looked first at the diet of the patient. Many of the plants in this book are foods: almonds, apples, dates, figs, mulberry, olives, pine nuts, pomegranates, asparagus, celery, garlic and grapes, all of which have wonderful medicinal properties, provided that they've been grown without pesticides. Many others, such as the culinary herbs: parsley, mint, rosemary, sage, bayleaves etc., also have powerful healing properties.

Ancient Greek doctors did not hesitate to tell their patients to change their diet, to include certain foods, to eliminate others and on occasion to eat less. They believed that two meals a day were sufficient for a slim person, while a fat person should limit themselves to one meal a day. Only after the subject of diet had been dealt with did they begin to prescribe herbal cures.

There is much that we can learn from this: we should consider that the food we eat will determine how healthy we can be. If we focus on foods which are good for us, such as vegetables, fruits, grains, pulses and nuts and try to avoid foods which are bad for us, above all sugar, which means avoiding all processed foods, we can improve our health immeasurably. Then and only then, we can start to use herbal medicines to treat any symptoms which still remain.

References

Introduction

Aegineta P Medical Compendium in 7 Books. Adams, 1844/1846/1847; Heiberg, 1921/1924.

Anneli S and Lawson R and K 1991. Goddess Sites: Europe. Harper Collins.

Alakbarov F 2003. Aromatic herbal baths of the ancients. Herbalgram 2003. 57: 40-49.

Apollodorus The library. Trans JG Frazer 1963-1967. Loeb Classical library Cambridge MA, Harvard Uni Press.

Apollonius Rhodius, Argonautica. Trans WH Race 2008. Loeb Classical Library 1. Cambridge MA and London: Harvard University Press.

Askitopoulou H et al 2002. Surgical cures under sleep induction in the Asclepieion of Epidauros. Internat Congress Series 1242 (2002): 11-17.

https://www.britannica.com/topic/Apollo-Greek-mythology

Corradini AM 1997. Meteres: Il Mito del matriarchato in Sicilia. 12-4; 81-3. Enna. Papiro.

Dioscorides De Materia Medica. Trans TA Osbaldeston and RPA Wood. Ibidis Press 2000.

Encyclopaedia Britannica. Pedanius Dioscorides Greek Physician.

Encyclopaedia Britannica. Crateuas Greek Artist and physician.

Encyclopaedia Britannica. Herbal Manual.

www.britannica.com/biography/Hippocrates Greek Physician: Wesley D. Smith.

Flaccus Valerius Argonautica. Trans JH Mozley Harvard Uni Press 1934.

Galen. Epidemiae 6.4.7, 5. 308L.

Gimbutas M 1989. Language of the goddess. Harper and Row.

http://www.greekmedicine.net/mythology/apollo.html

Hesiod 730-700 BCE. Theogony Trans HG Evelyn-White 2017 by

Createspace Independent Publishing Platform.

Hippocrates Corpus Hippocraticum. Henderson J ed. Trans Loeb Vols 1-4 1923–1931 Heinemann London. Loeb Vols 5-10 1988 - 2012 Harvard Uni Press.

Homer Odyssey. Trans P Green. 2018 Uni California Press.

Homer Illiad. Trans P Green 2015. Uni California Press.

Luck G 1985. Arcana Mundi. Magic and the Occult in the Greek and Roman Worlds. A Collection of ancient texts translated and Annotated and introduced by Georg Luck. John Hopkins Uni. Press, Baltimore.

March J 1998 Cassell's Dictionary of Classical Mythology. Cassell and Co. UK

Entry on Apollo - pg. 110.

Marinatos N 2000. Goddess and the Warrior. Routledge London NY.

https://www.mercatornet.com/articles/view/i_swear_by_apollo_the_healer/9491

Mariolakos E 2009. Geomythotopoi, p. 5.

Nutton V 2004. Ancient Medicine. Routledge.

Oberhelman SM 2014. Anatomical Votive reliefs as evidence for specialisation at healing sanctuaries in the ancient mediterranean word. Athens J Health1 (1): 47-62.

Pain S 2008. Histories: Mithridates's marvellous medicine. New Scientist 23 Jan 2008.

Pausanias Trans WHS Jones 1918. Vol I: Books 1-2 (Attica and Corinth). Loeb Classical Library 93. Cambridge, MA: Harvard University Press.

Pindar Pythian Odes. Trans WH Race 1997. Loeb Classical Library 56.

Plato Critias 4. 111. Loeb Classical Library 2020. Harvard Uni Press.

Pliny Natural History. Trans H Rackham vols 1-5, 9 WHS Jones vols 6-8 and DE Eichholz vol 10. London: Heinemann; Cambridge, Mass: Harvard University Press, 1938-1963.

Rigolioso M 2009. The cult of the divine birth in ancient Greece. Palgrave Macmillan.

Slattery DP 2018. The road from disease to recovery. A bio-mythic narrative.

Sophocles 497-406 BCE. Rhizotomoi.

Sophocles, Antigone, Trans R Gibbons C Segal 2003. Oxford Uni Press.

Theophrastus. Historia Plantarum. Trans Sir Arthur Hort 1916 Loeb Classical Library.

Van der Eijk ed Ancient Medicine in its socio-cultural context. Papers read at the congress held at Leiden University 13-15 April 1992 Vol 1.

Van der Molen The language of Asclepius. The role and diffusion of the written word in - and the visual language of - the cult of Asclepius 2019. University of Groningen.

Sacred Trees in Ancient Greece

Athenaeus Deipnosophists. Trans C.B. Gulick 1927-1930.

Oak Valonia

Anneli S and Lawson R and K 1991. Goddess Sites in Europe. Harper Collins.

Aristophanes. The complete plays. Trans Paul Roche. New American Library 2005.

Anneli S and Lawson R and K. Goddess Sites: Europe pub 1991.

Antoninus Liberalis. The Metamorphoses. Trans Francis Celoria. Routledge 1992.

Apollodorus The library. Trans JG Frazer 1963-1967. Loeb Classical Library Cambridge MA, Harvard Uni Press.

Apollonius Rhodius Argonautica. Trans WH Race 2008. Loeb Classical Library 1. Cambridge MA and London: Harvard University Press.

Athenaeus. Deipnosophistai ("The Gastronomers") Trans. C.D. Yonge 1854.

Homer Illiad. Trans P Green 2015. Uni California Press.

Gimbutas M 1989. Language of the goddess. Harper and Row.

Harrison JE 1913. Ancient art and ritual. Kessinger Publishing, 1995.

Harrison JE 1912. Themis: A Study of the social origins of Greek Religion.

Hesiod Works and Days. Trans HG Evelyn-White 1970 by Createspace Independent Publishing Platform.

Hesiod, Catalogues of Women Fragment 97 (from Scholiast on Sophocles Trachinae 1167): trans. Evelyn-White.

Herodotus The Histories: trans Tom Holland. Penguin Classics 2003.

Hesiod Homeric Hymns, Epic Cycle, Homerica. Trans Hugh C Evelyn-White Cambridge: Harvard Uni Press 1936.

Homer Iliad 16.235 trans Peter Green 2015 Univ of California Press.

Hunter R ed 2008 The Hesiodic Catalogue of Women. Constructions and Reconstructions. Cambridge University Press.

Kerenyi K. 1980. The Gods of the Greeks. Thames and Hudson.

Kerenyi K 1997. The Heroes of the Greeks. Thames and Hudson.

Levi P. 2012. Virgil: A Life. Bloomsbury Pub.

Pausanius Guide to Greece vol 1 central Greece VII. 21.1 p 281 trans SE Alcock, JE Cherry, J Elsner. Oxford Uni Press 2003.

Pausanias, Guide to Greece vol VII. 17. 8 trans. SE Alcock, JE Cherry, J Elsner. Oxford Uni Press 2003.

Philpot JH 1897. The Sacred Tree: or, the Tree in Religion and Myth. Macmillan.

Plato, Phaedrus 275b. Trans A Nehamas and Paul Woodruff. Hackett 1995.

Pliny the elder: A selection. Trans JF Healy. Penguin 1991.

Rigolioso M: The Cult of Divine Birth. Palgrave Macmillan 2009.

http://www.sacredthreads.net/www.sacredthreads.net/oak_at_ dodona.html

Sophocles works trans Robert Fagles. Penguin.

Strabo, Geography 5. 2. 4. Trans. Jones.

Strabo Geography 7 Fragment 1c trans Levi P. 1980. Atlas of the Greek World.

Stratton HF 1937. Dodona Privately printed in Philadelphia. https://www.theoi.com/Cult/ZeusDodonaiosCult.html

Valerius Flaccus Argonautica. Trans Andrew Zissos. Oxford Uni Press 2008.

Almond tree

Abdulla MK et al 2017. Badam (Prunus amygdalus Bail.): a fruit with medicinal properties. Int J Herbal Med 5 (5): 114-117.

Berryman CE et al 2017. Inclusion of almonds in a cholesterol-lowering diet improves plasma HDL subspecies and cholesterol efflux to serum in normal-weight individuals with elevated LDL cholesterol. J. Nutr. 147 (8) 1517 -1523.

Jenkins DJA et al 2008. Effect of almonds on insulin secretion and insulin resistance in non diabetic hyperlipidemic subjects. A randomised controlled crossover trial. Metab. Clan Exp 57: 882-887

Li N et al 2007. Almond consumption reduces oxidative stress in smokers. J. Nutr 2007; 137: 2717-2722.

Pausanias Trans WHS Jones 1918. Vol I: Books 1-2 (Attica and Corinth). Loeb Classical Library 93. Cambridge, MA: Harvard University Press.

Rajaram S et al 2009. Effect of almond-enriched high-monounsaturated fat diet on selected markers of inflammation: a randomised, controlled, crossover study. Br J Nutr 2009.

Sang S et al 2002. Antioxidative phenolic compounds isolated from almond skins (Prunus amygdalus Batsch). J Agric Food Chem 50 (8), 2459-2463.

Wijeratne SSK et al 2006. Antioxidant polyphenols in almond and its co-products. J Agric Food Chem. 54 (2), 312-318.

Yi M et al 2014. The effect of almond consumption on elements of endurance exercise performance in trained athletes. J. Int. Soc. Sports. Nutr 2014; 11:18.

Apple tree

Apollodorus The library. Trans JG Frazer 1963-1967. Loeb Classical library Cambridge MA, Harvard Uni Press.

Aprikian O et al 2001. Apple favourably affects parameters of cholesterol metabolism and of anti-oxidative protection in cholesterol fed rats. Food Chem. 2001; 75: 445-452.

Aprikian O et al 2003. Apple pectin and a polyphenol rich apple concentrate are more effective together than separately on cecal fermentations and plasma lipids in rats. J Nutr 2003; 133: 1860-1865.

Boyer J and Liu RH 2004 Apple phytochemicals and their health benefits. Nutri J 2004; 3: 5.

Breinholt V et al 2003. Effects of commonly consumed fruit juices and carbohydrates on redox status and anticancer biomarkers in female rats. Nutr Cancer 2003; 45: 46-52.

De Oliviera MC et al 2003. Weight loss associated with a daily intake of 3 apples or 3 pears among overweight women. Nutr. 2003; 19: 253-256.

De Silva P et al 2003. Antioxidant protection of low density lipoprotein by procyanidins: structure/activity relationships. Biochem Pharmacy. 66: 947-954.

Eberhardt M et al 2000. Antioxidant activity of fresh apples. Nature 2000. 405: 903-904.

Feskanich D et al 2000. Prospective study of fruit and vegetable consumption and risk of lung cancer among men and women. J Natl Cancer Inst. 2000; 92: 1812-1823. Hertog M et al 1993. Dietary antioxidant flavonoid and risk of coronary heart disease; The Zutphen Elderly Study. Lancet 1993; 342: 1007-1111.

Knekt P et al 2002. Flavonoid intake and risk of chronic diseases.

Am J Clin Nutr 2002. 76; 560-568.

Shaheen S et al 2001. Dietary antioxidants and asthma in adults - population based case-control study. Am J Respir Crit Care Med 2001; 164: 1823-1828.

Sun J et al 2002. Antioxidant and anti-proliferative activities of common fruits. J Agric Food Chem 2002. 50: 7449-7454.

Wolfe K et al 2003. Antioxidant activity of apple peels. J Agric food Chem 51 (3); 609-614.

Woods R et al 2003. Food and nutrient intakes and asthma risk in young adults. Am J Clin Nutr 2003; 78: 414-421.

Ash manna

Brown D 1995. Encyclopaedia of herbs and their uses. Dorling Kindersley, London.

Hendrick UP 1972. Sturtevant's Edible Plants of the World. Dover Pub.

Hesiod 730-700 BCE. Theogony. Trans HG Evelyn-White 2017 by Createspace Independent Publishing Platform.

Hill AF 1952. Economic Botany. The Maple Press.

Kissufiva T et al 2002. Escuside, a new coumarin-secoiridoid from *Fraxinus ornus* bark.

Kostova IN et al 1993. Secoiridoid and phenolic compounds from *Fraxinus ornus*.

Kostova IN and Iossifova T 2002. Studies in Natural Products Chemistry. Vol 26, Part G 313-349. Marinova EM et al 1994. Antioxidative action of the ethanol extract and hydroxycoumarins of *Fraxinus ornus* bark. Plants Medica 1993. 59; (S1); A705-A705.

TIossifova B et al 2002. Escuside, a new coumarin-secoiridoid from Fraxinus ornus bark. Fitoterapia 773 (5); 386-389.

Uphof JC 1959. Dictionary of Economic Plants Weinheim.

Wood G and Bache E. 1878.The Dispensatory of the United States of America, 14th edition (Philadelphia: Lippincott, 1878), pp. 572-575.

Chaste tree

Dericks-Tan J et al 2003. Dose-dependent stimulation of melatonin secretion after administration of Agnus castus. Experimental and clinical endocrinology and diabetes. 111: 44-46.

Dioscorides, De materia medica, I. 103. Trans Beck. 74.

Eftekhari MH et al 2014. Effects of Vitex agnus castus extract and magnesium supplementation, alone and in combination, on osteogenic factors and fracture healing in women with long bone fracture. J Res Med Sci 19 (1); 1-7.

Tesch BJ 2003. Herbs commonly used by women: an evidence based review. Am J Obstet Gynecol. https://doi.org/10.1067/mob.2003.402

Csupor D et al 2019. Vitex agnus-castus in premenstrual syndrome: A meta-analysis of double-blind randomised controlled trials. Complement Ther Med. 47; 102190.

Hughs K and Talbott SM 2006. The Health Professional's Guide to Dietary Supplements. Uppincott Williams and Wilkins.

Jazani M et al 2019. A comprehensive review of clinical studies with herbal medicine on polycystic ovary syndrome.

Pausanius. Guide to Greece. 2. 3. 4. Trans WHS Jones, 1: 261.

Pliny. Natural History. 24. 38. 62. Trans WHS Jones 7: 47.

Pliny, Natural History, 24. 38. 59. Trans WHS Jones, 7: 47.

Snow, JM 1996. Vitex agnus-castus L. (Verbenaceae) Protocol Journal. Herb clip 120262-101. American Botanical Council.

Stojkovic D et al 2011. Chemical composition and anti-microbial activity of Vitex agnus-castus L. fruits and leaves essential oils. Food chemistry 128 (4) 1017 - 1022.

Van Die MD et al 2009. Vitex agnus-castus (chaste-tree/berry) in the treatment of menopause-related complaints. J Altern Complement Med. 15(8): 853-862.

Von Staden trans. 29, based on text, Galen, *De simpl. med. temp. fac.*, 6. 2. Kühn ed., 11:807–808.

Von Staden. 38.

Wuttke W et al 2003. Chaste tree (Vitex agnus-castus) - Pharmacology and clinical indications Phytomedicine. 2003;10:348-357.

Cherry tree Cornelian

Alavian SM et al 2014. Protective effect of *Cornus mas* fruits extract on serum biomarkers in CCl4-induced hepatotoxicity in male rats. Hepat. Mon. 2014, 14, e10330.

Asgary S et al 2013. Investigation of the lipid-modifying and anti-inflammatory effects of *Cornus mas* L. supplementation on dyslipidemic children and adolescents. Pediatric Cardiology 34; 1729-1735.

Asquary S 2014. Biochemical and histopathological study of the anti-hyperglycemic and anti-hyperlipidemic effects of cornelian cherry (*Cornus mas* L.) in alloxan-induced diabetic rats. *J. Complement. Integr. Med.* 11, 63–69.

Athenaeus. Deipnosophistai ("The Gastronomers") Trans CD Yonge 1854.

Deng S 2013. UPLC-TOF-MS Characterization and Identification of Bioactive Iridoids in Cornus mas Fruit. Chem Med Plants, Foods, and Nat Prods. Volume 2013 | Article ID 710972 | 7 pages.

Dinda B et al 2016. Cornus mas L (cornelian cherry), an important European and Asian traditional food and medicine: Ethnomedicine, phytochemistry and pharmacology for its commercial utilisation in drug industry. J Ethnopharmacol. 193; 670-690.

He LH 2011. Comparative study for α-glucosidase inhibitory effects of total iridoid glycosides in the crude products and the wine-processed products from *Cornus officinalis*. Yakugaku Zasshi 131, 1801–1805.

Hosseinpour-Jaghdani F et al 2017. Cornus mas: a review on traditional uses and pharmacological properties. J Complement Integr Med. 14; 3. https://doi.org/10.1515/jcim-

2016-0137.

Kyriakopoulos AM and Dinda B 2006. *Cornus mas* (Linnaeus) Novel devised medicinal preparations: bactericidal effect against *Staphylococcus aureus* and *Pseudomonas aeruginosa*. Molecules 20 (6): 11202-11218.

Petridis A et al 2010. Antioxidant activity of fruits produced in northern Greece. Hortscience 45, 1341–1344.

Skinner CM 1911. Myths and Legends of Flowers, Trees, Fruits and Plants. Read Books.

Soltani R et al 2015. Evaluation of the effects of Cornus mas L fruit extract on glycemic control and insulin level in type 2 diabetic adult patients: a randomised double-blind placebo-controlled clinical trial. Evid Based Complement Alt Med. published online https://doi.org/10.1155/2015/740954

Fig tree

Athenaeus. Deipnosophistai ("The Gastronomers") Trans CD Yonge 1854.

Atkinson FS et al 2019. Abscisic acid standardised fig (Ficus carica) extracts ameliorate postprandial glycemic and insulinemic responses in healthy adults. Nutrients 11: 1757.

Bahadori et al 2016. A study of the effect of an oral formulation of fig and olive on rheumatoid arthritis remission indicators: A randomised clinical trial. Iranian J Pharm Res 15 (3): 537-545.

Brussell DE 2005. Medicinal plants of Mt Pelion, Greece. Econ Bot 58 (Supplement) S174-S202.

Homer Illiad. Trans P Green 2015. Uni California Press.

Canal JR et al 2000. Chloroform extract obtained from a decoction of Ficus carica leaves improves the cholesterolaemic status of rats with streptozotocin-induced diabetes. Acta Physiologica Hungarica 87, 71-76.

Conduit I. 1955. Fig varieties: a monograph. Hilgardia. 23 (11): 323-538.

Duke 1992. Handbook of Phytochemical constituents of GRAS herbs and other economic plants. CRC Press, Boca Raton USA pp 117-118.

Fulani A et al 2008 Ethnopharmacological studies on anti-spasmodic and anti platelet activities of Ficus carica. J ethnophrmacol 119 (1); 1-5.

Fuller DQ and Stevens CJ 2019. Between domestication and civilisation: the role of agriculture and arboriculture in the emergence of the first urban societies. Veget Hist Archeobot 28: (3): 263-282.

Jeong MR et al 2009. Anti-microbial activity of methanol extract from Ficus carica leaves against oral bacteria. J Bacterol and Virol 39 (2); 97-102.

Lansky EP and Paavilainen HM eds 2011. Figs: the Genus Ficus. Boca Raton FL: CRC Press.

Patil VV et al 2010. Evaluation of anti-pyretic potential of Ficus carica leaves. Internat J Pharmaceut Sciences Rev and Res 2 (2); 48-50.

Pausanias Trans WHS Jones 1918. Vol I: Books 1-2 (Attica and Corinth). Loeb Classical Library 93. Cambridge, MA: Harvard University Press.

Penelope O 1997. 100 Great Natural Remedies. Kyle Cathic Limited, New York pp 98-99.

Pourmasoumi M et al 2019. Comparison and assessment of flixweed and fig effects on irritable bowel syndrome with predominant constipation: A single-blind randomised clinical trial. EXPLORE 15 (3): 487-496.

Richter G 2002. Activation and inactivation of human factor X by proteases derived from Ficus carica. British J Haematol 119, 1042-1051.

Sardari M et al 2015. Ficus carica fig paste supplementation in patients with multiple sclerosis associated constipation: a double blind, randomised clinical trial. Planta med. 81: (16): SI. 2A.04.

Shukranul M et al 2013. Ficus carica L (Moraceae): Phytochemistry, traditional uses and biological activities. Evidence-based complementary and alternative medicine. Article ID 974256, 8 pages. http://dx.doi.org/10.1155/2013/974256.

Solomon A et al 2006. Antioxidant activities and anthocyanin content of fresh fruits of common fig (Ficus carica L). J Agric Food Chem 20, 7717-7723.

Tofighi Z et al 2017. Formulation and evaluation of an Iranian traditional dosage form containing Linum and Ficus for improvements of functional constipation. Jundishapur J Nat Pharm Prod 12 (4): e40069.

Frankincense tree

Bongers F 2019. Frankincense in peril. Nature Sustainability 2; 602-610.

Gerhardt H 2001.Therapy of active Crohn disease with Boswellia serrata extract H 15. Zeitschrift fur Gastroenterologie, 01 Jan 2001, 39(1):11-17.

Doaee 2019 Effects of Boswellia serrata resin extract on motor dysfunction and brain oxidative stress in an experimental model of Parkinson's disease. Avicenna J Phytomed. 9 (3); 281-290.

Gupta I et al 1997. Effects of Boswellia serrata gum resin in patients with ulcerative colitis. European Journal of Medical Research, 01 Jan 1997, 2(1):37-43.

Murray MT. Rocklin, CA: 1995. The Healing Power of Herbs; Prima Publishing; pp. 327–35.

Ovid The Metamorphoses. Trans AS Kline 2000. Pan American.

Poeckel D Werz O 2006. Current Medicinal Chemistry 13 (28); 3359-3369

Rall B et al 1996. Boswellic acids and protease activities. Phytomed. 3:75–6.

Shishodia et al 2008. The guggul for chronic diseases: ancient medicine, modern targets. Anticancer Res. 28, 3647–3664.

Singh GB, Atal CK. 1984. Pharmacology of an extract of salai guggul ex- Boswellia serrata. Indian J Pharmacol. 16:51.

Singh HP et al 2012. In vitro antioxidant and free radical scavenging activity of different extracts of Boerhavia diffusa and Boswellia serrata. Int J Pharma Sci Res. 2012;3:503–511.

Laurel or sweet bay

Afifi FU et al 1997. Evaluation of the gastroprotective effect of Laurus nobilis seeds on ethanol induced gastric ulcer in rats. Journal of Ethnopharmacology. 58: 9-14.

Corato DU, et al 2007. Anti-fungal activity of the leaf extracts of laurel (Laurus nobilis L.), orange (Citrus sinensis Osbeck) and olive (Olea europaea L.) obtained by means of supercritical carbon dioxide technique. Journal of Plant Pathology. 89 (3): 83-91.

Elmastas M et al 2006. Radical Scavenging Activity and Antioxidant Capacity of Bay Leaf Extracts. Journal of the Iranian Chemical Society. 3(3): 258-266.

Erler F et al 2006. Repellent activity of 5 essential oils against Culex pipiens. Fitoterapia. 77 (7-8): 491-494.

Ferreira A et al 2006. The in vitro screening for acetylcholinesterase inhibition and antioxidant activity of medicinal plants from Portugal. Journal of Ethnopharmacol. 108 (1): 31-37.

Ham A, et al 2011. Neuroprotective Effect of the n- Hexane Extracts of Laurus nobilis L. in Models of Parkinson's Disease. Biomol Ther. 19(1): 118-125.

Loizzo MR et al 2008. Phytochemical analysis and in vitro anti-viral activities of the essential oils of 7 Lebanon species. Chem Biodivers. 5 (3): 461-470.

Macchioni F et al 2006. Composition and acaricidal activity of Laurus novocanariensis and Laurus nobilis essential oils against Psoroptes cuniculi. Journal of Essential Oil Research. 18: 111-114.

Nayak S et al 2006. Evaluation of wound healing activity of

Allamanda cathartica. L. and Laurus nobilis. L. extracts on rats. Complementary and Alternative Medicine. 2006; 6: 12.

Ovid The Metamorphoses. Trans AS Kline 2000. Pan American.

Ozcan B et al 2010. Effective anti-bacterial and antioxidant properties of methanolic extract of Laurus nobilis seed oil. Journal of Environmental Biology. 31(5): 637-64.

Patrakar R et al 2012. Phytochemical and pharmacological review on Laurus nobilis. Internat J pharmaceutical and chemical sciences ISSN: 2277-5005.

Samejima K et al 1998. Bay Laurel Contains Anti-mutagenic kaempferyl coumarate acting against the dietary carcinogen 3-Amino-1-methyl-5H-pyrido (4, 3- blindole.) J. Agric. Food Chem. 46 (12): 4864–4868.

Sayyah M et al 2003. Analgesic and anti- inflammatory activity of the leaf essential oil of Laurus nobilis Linn. Phytotherapy Research. 17 (7): 733–736.

Sayyah M et al 2002. Anticonvulsant activity of the leaf essential oil of Laurus nobilis against pentylenetetrazole and maximal electroshock-induced seizures. Phytomed. 9: 212-216.

Lime or Linden

Anesini C et al 1999. Effect of *Tilia cordata* flower on lymphocyte proliferation: Participation of peripheral type benzodiazepine binding sites. Fitoterapia 70 (4): 361-367.

Barnes J et al 2007. Herbal Medicines. 2 ed. Pharmaceutical Press, London; 409-410.

Blumenthal M et al editors. 1998. The Complete German Commission E Monographs. "Linder flower – *Tiliae flos*". American Botanical Council, Austin Texas 1998, 163.

Blumenthal M et al editors. 2000. Herbal Medicine Expanded Commission E Monographs. American Botanical Council, Austin Texas 240-243.

Bradley P, ed. 1992. British Herbal Compendium. Vol. I. Dorset (Great Britain): British Herbal Medicine Association: 142-144.

European Medicines Agency 2012. Committee on Herbal Medicinal Products (HMPC) Assessment report on *Tilia cordata* Miller, *Tilia platyphyllos* Scop., *Tilia x vulgaris* Heyne or their mixtures, *flos* EMA/HMPC/337067/2011.

Guerin JC and Reveillere HP 1984. Anti-fungal activity of plant extracts used in therapy. I. Study of 41 plant extracts against 9 fungi species. Ann. Pharm. Fr. B: 553–559. [in French: Activité antifongique d'extraits végétaux à usage thérapeutique. I. Etude de 41 extraits sur 9 souches fongiques.

Hyginus GJ Fabulae trans Mary Grant 1960.

Lanza JP, Steinmetz M. Actions comparées des extraits aqueux de graines de *Tilia platyphylla* et de *Tilia vulgaris* sur l'intestin isolé de rat. [Comparison of actions of aqueous extracts of *Tilia platyphylla* and *Tilia vulgaris* seeds on isolated rat intestine]. Fitoterapia 1986, 57: 185.

Nowak R 2003. Separation and quantification of tiliroside from plant extracts by SPE/RP-HPLC. Pharm. Biology 41(8): 627-630.

Otoom SA et al 2006. The use of medicinal herbs by diabetic Jordanian patients. J. Herbal Pharmacother; 6 (2): 31-41.

Ovid The Metamorphoses. Trans AS Kline 2000. Pan American.

Ranilla LG et al 2010. Phenolic compounds, antioxidant activity and *in vitro* inhibitory potential against key enzymes relevant for hyperglycemia and hypertension of commonly used medicinal plants, herbs and spices in Latin America. Biores. Technol. 101(12): 4676-4689.

Taddei I et al 1988. Spasmolytic activity of peppermint, sage and rosemary essences and their major constituents. Fitoterapia 59: 463–468.

Viola H et al 1994. Isolation of pharmacologically active benzodiazepine receptor ligands from *Tilia tomentosa* (Tiliaceae). J. Ethnopham. 44: 47–53.

WHO 2010 monographs on medicinal plants commonly used in the Newly Independent States (NIS). *"Tiliae flos"*. Geneva,

Switzerland 2010, 393-406.

Zhang Z-J 2004. Therapeutic effects of herbal extracts and constituents in animal models of psychiatric disorders. Life Sciences 75(14): 1659-1699.

Lotus tree or Date Plum

Chopra RN et al 1992. Glossary of Indian. Medicinal Plants. 3rd edition. CSIR. New Delhi 99.

Gao H 2014. Antioxidant activities and phenolic compounds of date plum persimmon (*Diospyros lotus* L.) fruits. Journal of Food Science and Technology. 51 (5); 950–956.

Gul H et al 2014. Phytochemical analysis and biological activities of *Diospyros lotus* L. fruit extracts. International Journal of Pharmaceutical Chemistry.

Herath WW et al 1978 'Triterpenoid, coumarin and quinone constituents of eleven *Diospyros species* (Ebenaceae)', Phytochemistry, 17(5), 1007-1009.

Homer Odyssey IX trans P Green 2015. Uni California Press.

Khaled Rashed, Xing-Jie Zhang, Meng-Ting Luo, Yang-Tang Zheng, Anti-HIV-1 activity of phenolic compounds isolated from *Diospyros lotus* fruits, Phytopharmacology 2012, 3(2) 199-207.

Ovid The Metamorphoses. Trans AS Kline 2000. Pan American.

Pant S and Samant SS 2010. Ethanobotanical observation in the Momaula Reserve Forest of Koumoun West Himalaya, India. Ethnobotanical Leaflets 1493.

Rauf A et al 2015. A rare class of new dimeric naphthoquinones from Diospyros lotus have multi drug reversal and anti proliferative effects. Front. Pharmacol; 16 Dec 2015. https://doi.org/10.3389/fphar.2015.00293

Rauf et al 2015. *In vivo* sedative and muscle relaxant activity of *Diospyros lotus* L. Asian Pacific Journal of Tropical Biomedicine. 5 (4); 277-280.

Rauf et al 2017. Sedative-hypnotic-like effect and molecular docking of di-naphthodiospyrol from *Diospyros lotus* in an animal model. Biomedicine and Pharmacotherapy 88: 109-113.

Sharma V 2017. Brief Review on the Genus *Diospyros*: A Rich Source of Naphthoquinones. Asian J. Adv. Basic Sci. 5 (2); 34-53.

Watt JM, Breyer-Brandwijk MG (1932) The Medicinal and Poisonous Plants of South Africa. Postgrad Med J 8: 427.

Ray, S et al 1998. Diospyrin, a bisnaphthoquinone: a novel inhibitor of type I DNA topoisomerase of *Leishmania donovani*', Molecular pharmacology, 54(6), 994-999.

Waterman P G and Mbi CN 1979. The sterols and dimeric naphthoquinones of the barks of 3 West Africa *Diospyros species* Planta Medica, 37 (11), 241-246.

Mulberry

Andallu B and Varadacharyulu NC 2003. Antioxidant role of mulberry *(Morus indica* L. cv. Anantha) leaves in streptozotocin-diabetic rats. Clin Chim Acta; 338: 3-10.

Asano N, et al 2001. Polyhydroxylated alkaloids isolated from mulberry trees (*Morus alba* L.) and silkworms (Bombix mori L.). J Agric Food Chem 49: 4208-13.

Chang JJ et al 2013. Mulberry anthocyanin inhibit oleic acid induced lipid accumulation by reduction of lipogenesis and promotion of hepatic lipid clearance. J Agric Chem 26; 61 (25): 6069

Chang LW et al 2011. Antioxidant and antityrosinase activity of mulberry (*Morus alba* L.) twigs and root bark. Food Chem Toxicol. 49: 785-90.

Chen PN et al 2006. Mulberry anthocyanins, cyanidin 3-rutinoside and cyanidin 3- glucoside, exhibited an inhibitory effect on the migration and invasion of a human lung cancer cell line. Cancer Lett. 235: 248-59.

Doi K et al 2000. Mulberry leaf extract inhibits the oxidative modification of rabbit and human low density lipoprotein. Biol Pharm Bull 2000; 23: 1066-71.

Harauma A, et al 2007. Mulberry leaf powder prevents atherosclerosis in apolipoprotein E-deficient mice. Biochem Biophys Res Commun. 358: 751-6.

Iyengar MNS 2007. Research Beliefs. Indian silk, July, 29.

Khaengkhan P et al 2009. Identification of an antiamyloidogenic substance from mulberry leaves. Neuroreport. 20: 1214-8.

Kim AJ and Park S 2006. Mulberry extract supplements ameliorate the inflammation-related hematological parameters in carrageenan-in-duced arthritic rats. J Med Food. 9: 431-5.

Kojima Y et al 2010. Effects of mulberry leaf extract rich in 1-deoxynojirimycin on blood lipid profiles in humans. J Clin Biochem Nutr 2010; 47: 155-61.

Kumar VR 2008. Mulberry: Life enhancer. Journal of Medicinal Plants Research 2(10), pp. 271-278.

Liu LK et al 2008. Mulberry anthocyanin extracts inhibit LDL oxidation and macrophage-derived foam cell formation induced by oxidative LDL. J Food Sci 73 (6): H113-21.

Masilamani S et al 2008. Mulberry fruits: A potential value - addition enterprise. Indian silk. 46(11):12.

Naowaboot J et al 2009. Antihyperglycemic, antioxidant and antiglycation activities of mulberry leaf extract in streptozotocin-induced chronic diabetic rats. Plant Foods Hum Nutr. 64: 116–21.

Ovid The Metamorphoses. Trans AS Kline 2000. Pan American.

Sanshi Shikenjo Iho. Technical Bull of Sericultural Experiment Station. 59; 9.

Scrivastava S et al 2003. Mulberry (*Morus alba*) leaves as human food: a new dimension in sericulture. Int J Food Sci Nutr 2003; 338: 3-10.

Sener B and Binjol F 1988. Int. J Crude Drug Research. 26:197.

Shivkumar GR et al 1995. Indian silk. 34:5.

Singh KP and Ghosh PL 1992. Indian silk. 31:16.

Sulochana P 2012. Medicinal Values of Mulberry - An Overview. J Pharm Res 5 (7); 3588-3596.

Suzuki B and Sakuma T 1941. On the Hypotensive components of the Mulberry tree.

Ting-Tsz O et al 2011. Mulberry extract inhibits oleic acid-induced lipid accumulation via reduction of lipogenesis and promotion of hepatic lipid clearance. Sci Food Agric 91 915): 2740-8

Zhang X et al 2009b. Inhibitory effect of 2,4,2',4'- tetrahydroxy-3-(3-methyl-2-butenyl)-chalcone on tyrosinase activity and melanin biosynthesis. Biol Pharm Bull. 32: 86- 90.

Myrrh tree

Albishri J 2017. The efficacy of myrrh in oral ulcer in patients with Behcet's Disease. American Journal of Research Communication, 2017, 5 (1): 23-28.

Arora RB et al 1973 Ind. J. Exp. Biol. 11, 166; C. A. 81, 109.

Atta AH 1998 Anti-nociceptive and anti-inflammatory effects of some Jordanian medicinal plant extracts. J Ethnopharmacol 60; 117.

Al Harbi MM et al 1997. Gastric anti-ulcer and cytoprotective effect of *Commiphora molmol* in rats. J. Ethnopharmacol. 55 (2): 141-150.

Al Awadi FM and Gumaa KA 1987. Studies on the activity of individual plants of an antidiabetic plant mixture. Acta Diabetol. Lat. 24, 37.

Al Awadi FM et al 1991. The effect of a plant's mixture extract on liver gluconeogenesis in streptozotocin induced diabetic rats. Diabetes Res. 18, 163.

Apollodorus The library. Trans JG Frazer 1963-1967. Loeb Classical library Cambridge MA, Harvard Uni Press.

Bailly C 2020. Xihuang pills, a traditional Chinese preparation used as a complementary medicine to treat cancer: An updated review. World J Trad Chinese Medicine. 6 (2): 152-

162.

Bown D 1995. Encyclopedia of Herbs and their Uses. Dorling Kindersley.

Chevallier A 1996. The Encyclopedia of Medicinal Plants. Dorling Kindersley.

Dioscorides P. De Materia Medica Lib 1, cap l xviij.

Dolara P et al 2000. Planta Med. 66, 356.

El Ashry 2003. Components, therapeutic value and uses of myrrh. Pharmazie 58: 163–168.

El-Sherbiny GM and El-Sherbiny ET 2011. The Effect of *Commiphora molmol* (Myrrh) in Treatment of *Trichomoniasis vaginalis* infection. Iran Red Crescent Med J. 13 (7): 480-486.

Jain SK 1994. Ethnobotany and research in medicinal plants in India. Ciba Found. Symp. 185, 153.

Kubec, F et al 1988. Czech. CS Pat. 244387; C.A. 109; 236732.

Lata, S et al 1991. Beneficial effects of *Allium sativum*, *Allium cepa* and *Commiphora mukul* on experimental hyperlipidemia and atherosclerosis--a comparative evaluation. Postgrad. Med. 37, 132.

Lee TY and Lam TH 1993. Allergic contact dermatitis due to a Chinese orthopaedic solution Tieh Ta Yao Gin. Contact Dermatitis 28, 89.

Mao D, et al 2019. Meta-analysis of Xihuang pill efficacy when combined with chemotherapy for treatment of breast cancer. Evid Based Complement Alternat Med: 3502460.

Michie CA and Cooper E 1991. Frankincense and myrrh as remedies in children. J Roy Soc Med 84, 602.

Narain Sharma, J.; Nath Sharma, 1977. Comparison of the anti-inflammatory activity of *Commiphora mukul* (an indigenous drug) with those of phenylbutazone and ibuprofen in experimental arthritis induced by mycobacterial adjuvant.J.: Arzneim. Forsch. Drug Res. 27, 1455.

Olajide OA 1999. Investigation of the effects of selected medicinal plants on experimental thrombosis. Phytother Res

13; 231.

Pesko LJ 1990. Components, therapeutic value and uses of myrrh. Am. Drug. 202, 90; Int. Pharm. Abstr. 28, 4186.

Qureshi S et al 1993. Evaluation of the genotoxic, cytotoxic, and anti-tumor properties of Commiphora molmol using normal and Ehrlich ascites carcinoma cell-bearing Swiss albino mice. Cancer Chemother Pharmacol 33, 130.

Rashad A et al 2009. Myrrh and trematodoses in Egypt: An overview of safety, efficacy and effectiveness profiles. Parasitol Internat 58 (3): 210-214.

Sarbhoy AK et al 1978. Efficacy of some essential oils and their constituents on few ubiquitous molds. Zentralbl. Bakteriol. (Naturwiss.) 133, 723.

Trease GE and Evans WC 1989. Pharmacognosy 13th ed., 474.

Tripathi YB et al 1984. Thyroid stimulating action of Z-guggulsterone obtained from *Commiphora mukul*. Planta Med. 50, 78.

Wallis TE Ed. 1967. Text book of Pharmacognosy, 5th ed., 497.

Vander Zanden JA and Fitzpatrick RB 1980. Minn. Pharm. 35, 8. Int. Pharm. Abstr. 18, 1640.

Myrtle

Amensour M et al 2010. Antioxidant activity and total phenolic compounds of myrtle extracts, J Food, 8 (2), 95-101.

Al-Hindawi et al 1989. Anti-inflammatory activity of some Iraqi plants in intact rats. J Ethnopharmacol. 26 (2), 163-168.

Agarwal VS 1999. Economic Plants of India, Kailash Prakashan, Calcutta, 1986; 251.

Alem G et al 2008. *In vitro* anti-bacterial activity of crude preparation of myrtle (*Myrtus communis*) on common human pathogens, Ethiop Med J, 46 (1), 63-69.

Baitar ZI 1999. Aljameul Mufradat Al-advia-wa- al-Aghzia. Vol.1, Translated by CCRUM, New Delhi, 1999, pp. 42-47.

Babaee N et al 2010. The efficacy of a paste containing Myrtus communis (Myrtle) in the management of recurrent aphthous stomatitis: A randomized controlled trial. Clin Oral Invest. 14, 65-70.

Diaz AM and Abeger A 1987. Phenolic compounds of the seeds 54 of *Myrtus communis* L., Plant Med Phytother, 21(4), 317-322.

Dineel A S et al 2007. Effects of *in vivo* antioxidant enzyme activities of myrtle oil in normoglycemic and alloxan diabetic rabbits, J Ethnopharmacol. 110 (3), 498-503.

Elfellah M S et al 1984. Anti-hyperglycaemic effect of an extract of *Myrtus communis* in streptozotocin-induced diabetes in mice, J Ethnopharmacol, 11(3), 275-281.

Fahim A B et al 2009. Biochemical studies on the effect of phenolic compounds extracted from *Myrtus communis* in diabetic rats, Tamilnadu J Vet Anim Sci. 5(3), 87-93.

Feisst C, et al 2005. Identification of molecular targets of the oligomeric nonprenylated acylphloroglucinols from *Myrtus communis* and their implication as anti-inflammatory compounds, J Pharmacol Exp Ther, 315(1), 389-396.

Ghani M N 1920. Khazainul Advia, Sheikh Mohammad Bashir and Sons Publication, Urdu Bazar, Lahore, Vol. III; 444-445.

Hakeem MA, 1895. Bustanul Mufradat, Idara Tarraqui Urdu Publications, Lucknow. 278.

Hayder N et al 2008. *In vitro* antioxidant and antigenotoxic potentials of myricetin-3-O-galactoside and myricetin-3-O-rhamnoside from *Myrtus communis*: Modulation of expression of genes involved in cell defence system using DNA microarray. Toxicol *In Vitro*. 22(3) 567-581.

Kabiruddin M 1951. Makhzan-ul-Mufradat, Sheikh Mohammad Bashir and Sons, Lahore, Pakistan 47-48.

Kirtikar KR and Basu BD 1988. Indian Medicinal Plants, 3rd Edn, International Book Distributors, Dehra Dun, Vol. II, 1040-1042.

Masoudi M 2016. Comparison of the Effects of *Myrtus Communis*

L, Berberis Vulgaris and Metronidazole Vaginal Gel alone for the Treatment of Bacterial Vaginosis. Journal of Clinical and Diagnostic Research : JCDR 10 (3); QC04-QC07.

Mimica-Dukic N et al 2010. Essential oil of *Myrtus communis* L. as a potential antioxidant and anti-mutagenic agents. Molecules; 15 (4), 2759-2770.

Nadkarni K M, Indian Materia Medica, 3rd Edn,1989. Popular Prakashan Pvt. Ltd., Bombay, vol. 1, 838.

Rastogi R P and Mehrotra BN 1991. Compendium of Indian Medicinal Plants (1970-1979), Central Drug Research Institute Lucknow, Vol. 2, Publications and Information Directorate, CSIR, New Delhi; 478.

Rosa A et al 2008. Protective effect of the oligomeric acylphloroglucinols from *Myrtus communis* on cholesterol and human low density lipoprotein oxidation, Chem Phys Lipids. 155 (1), 16-23.

Salouage I et al 2009. Effect of *Myrtus communis* L. on an experimental model of a rat liver ischemia-reperfusion. International Symposium on Medicinal and Aromatic Plants, ISHS Acta Hortic. 853.

Serce S et al 2010. Antioxidant activities and fatty acid composition of wild grown myrtle (*Myrtus communis* L.) fruits, Phcog Mag, 6, 9-12.

Slimeni O et al 2017. Effect of *Myrtus communis* supplementation on anaerobic performance and selected serum biochemical parameters. Med dello Sport. 70:150–62.

Sumbul S et al 2010. Evaluation of Myrtus communis Linn. berries (common myrtle) in experimental ulcer models in rats, Hum Exp Toxicol. 29 (11), 935-944.

Sumbul S 2011. Myrtus communis Linn. - A Review. I J N P R 2 (4); 19.

Stuart M 1994. The Encyclopedia of Herbs and Herbalism, 3rd Edn. 52, 136.

Trease W and Evans D 2006. Pharmacognosy, 15th Edn, W.B.

Saunders Comp Ltd., Toronto.

Nadkarni K M 1989. Indian Materia Medica, 3rd Edn, Popular Prakashan Pvt. Ltd., Bombay, vol. 1; 838.

Zohalinezhad ME 2015. Myrtus communis L. Freeze-Dried Aqueous Extract Versus Omeprazol in Gastrointestinal Reflux Disease: A Double-Blind Randomized Controlled Clinical Trial. Journal of Evidence-Based Complementary & Alternative Medicine, Volume: 21 issue: 1, page(s): 23-29.

Olive tree

Al-Azzawie HF and Alhamdani MS 2006. Hypoclycemic and antioxidant effect of oleuropein in alloxan-diabetic rabbits. Life Sci 78: 1371-1377.

Al-Qarawi AA et al 2002. Effect of freeze dried extract of *Olea europaea* on the pituitary-thyroid axis in rats. Phytotherapy Res 16: 286-287.

Apollodorus The Library. Trans JG Frazer 1963-1967. Loeb Classical library Cabridge MA, Harvard Uni Press.

Benavent-Garcia O et al 2000. Antioxidant activity of phenolics extracted from *Olea europaea* L. Leaves. Food chem 68:457-462.

Bennani-Kabchi N et al 1999. Effects of *Olea europea var. oleaster* leaves in hyper-cholesterolemic insulin-resistant sand rats. Therapie 54 (6): 717-23.

Briante R et al 2002. *Olea europaea* L. Leaf extract and derivatives: antioxidant properties. J Agric Food Chem 50: 4934-4940.

Bisignano G et al 1999. On the *in-vitro* anti-microbial activity of oleuropein and hydroxytyrosol. J Pharm Pharmacol 51 (8): 971-974.

Caturla N 2005. Differential effects of oleuropein, a biophenol from *Olea europaea*, on anionic and zwiterionic phospholipid model membranes. Chem Phys Lipids 137: 2-17.

Capretti G and Bonaconza E 1949. Effect of infusion of decoctions of olive leaves (*Olea europaea*) on some physical constants of blood (viscosity and surface tension) and on some. Giorn Clin Med.

Chimi H et al 1995. Inhibition of iron toxicity in rat hepatocyte culture by natural phenolic compounds. Tox *in vitro* 9: 695-702.

Cruess WV 1915-1965 Papers.

De Bock M et al 2013. Olive (*Olea europaea* L.) leaf polyphenols improve insulin sensitivity in middle-aged overweight men: a randomised placebo-controlled, crossover trial. PloS one 8 (3), e57622.

De Nino L et al 2005. Absolute method for the assay of oleuropein in olive oils by atmospheric pressure chemical ionisation tandem mass spectrometry. Anal Chem 77: 5961-5964.

Gonzalez M et al 1992. Hypoglycemic activity of olive leaf. Planta Med 58: 513-515.

Hanbury D 1874. Pharmacographia Macmillan.

Hanbury D 1841. Trans Pharmaceut Soc. 1. London: J and A Churchill.

Hansen K et al 1996. Isolation of an angiotensin converting enzyme (ACE) inhibitor from *Olea europaea* and *Olea lacea*. Phytomedicine 2: 319-325.

Heinze JE et al 1975. Specificity of the anti-viral agent calcium elenolate. Anti-microbial Agents Chemother 8 (4): 421-5.

Shesh A 2005. The Herbs of Avurveda 3: 820.

Khan Y 2007. *Olea europaea*: A Phyto-Pharmacological Review. Pharmacog Rev 1 (1).

Susalit E 2011. Olive (*Olea europaea*) leaf extract effective in patients with stage-1 hypertension: Comparison with Captopril. Phytomed 18 (4): 251-258.

Kushi LH et al 1995. Health implications of Mediterranean diets in light of contemporary knowledge. Meat, wine, fats and oils. Am J Clin Nutr 61: 1416S-1427S.

Perrinjaquet-Moccetti T 2008. Food supplementation with an olive (*Olea europaea* L.) leaf extract reduces blood pressure in borderline hypertensive monozygotic twins. Phytother Res 22 (9): 1239-1242.

Petroni A et al 1995. Inhibition of platelet aggregation and eicosanoid production by phenolic components of olive oil. Thromb Res 78 (2): 151-160.

Petkov V and Manolov P 1972. Pharmacological analysis of the iridoid oleuropein. Drug Res 22 (9): 1476-86.

Pieroni A et al 1996. *In vitro* anti-complementary activity of flavonoids from olive (*Olea europaea* L) leaves. Pharmazie 51 (10): 765-768.

Renis HE 1970. *In vitro* anti-viral activity of calcium elenolate. Anti-microbial Agents Chemother 167-72.

Soret MC 1969. Anti-viral activity of calcium elenolate on parainfluenza infection of hamsters. Anti-microbial Agents and Chemother 9: 160-66.

Visioli F et al 1994. Oleuropein protects low density lipoprotein from oxidation. Life Sci 55: 71.

Visioli F et al 2002. Antioxidant and other biological activities of phenols from olives and olive oil. Med Res Rev 22: 65-75.

Weinstein J 2012. Olive leaf extract as a hypoglycaemic agent in both human diabetic subjects and in rats. J Med Food 15 (7).

Zarzuelo A et al 1991. Vasodilator effect of olive leaf. Planta Med. 57 (5): 417-9.

Zaslaver M et al 2005. Natural compounds derived from foods modulate nitric oxide production and oxidative status in epithelial lung cells. J Agric Food Chem., 53: 9934-9939.

Palm date

Al-Farsi et al 2005. Comparison of antioxidant activity, anthocyanin, carotenoids and phenolic of 3 native fresh and sun dried date (Phoenix dactylifera L.) varieties grown in Oman. J Agric and food chef 53: 7592-7599.

Allaith A 2005. In vitro evaluation of antioxidant activity of different extracts of Phoenix dactylifera L. Fruit as functional foods. Deutsche Lebensmittel Rundschau 101: 305-308.

Al-Taher AY 2008. Possible antidiarrhoeal effect of date-palm (Phoenix dactylifera L.) aqueous extracts in rats. Scientific J King Faisal Uni (Basic and Applied Sciences) 9; 1429-1435.

Al Qarawi AA et al 2003. Gastrointestinal transit in mice treated with various extracts of date (Phoenix dactylifera L.) Food Chem Toxicol 41; 37-39.

Al-Qarawi AA et al 2004. Protective effect of extracts of dates (Phoenix dactylifera L.) on carbon tetrachloride-induced hepatotoxicity in rats. Int J App Res Vet Med 2: 176-180.

Al-Qarawi AA et al 2005. The ameliorative effect of dates (Phoenix dactylifera L.) on ethanol induced gastric ulcer in rats. J Ethnopharmacol 98; 313-317.

Ayachi A et al 2009. Anti-bacterial activity of some fruits; berries and medicinal herb extracts against poultry strains of Salmonella. American-eurasian J Agic and Enviro Sci 6 (1), 12-15.

Duke JA and Wain KK 1981. Medicinal plants of the world. Computer index with more than 85,000 entries. 3 vols.

Elgasim EA et al 1995. Possible hormonal activity of date pits and flesh fed to meat animals. Food Chem 52; 149-150.

Homeric Hymns. trans Peter Green 2015 Univ of California Press.

Isruda O and John FK 2005. The anticancer activity of polysaccharide prepared from Libyab dates (Phoenix dactylifera L.) Carbohydrate Polymers 59; 531-535 (s).

Mohammed and Al-Okbi 2004. In vivo evaluation of antioxidant and anti-inflammatory activity of different extracts of date fruits in adjuvant arthritis. Polish J food nutrition Sci 13: 397-201.

Mohammed BA et al 2008. Protective effects of extracts from dates (Phoenix dactylifera L.) and ascorbic acid on thioacetamide-induced hepatotoxicity in rats. Iranian J Pharm Res 7; 193-201.

Nasiri M 2019. Effects of consuming date fruits (Phoenix

dactylifera Linn) on gestation, labor, and delivery: An updated systematic review and meta-analysis of clinical trials. Complementary Ther Med. 45; 71-84.

Panahi A and Asadi M 2009. Cholesterol lowering and protective effects of date fruit extracts: an in vivo study. Toxicology Letters 189S: S57-S273 (F25).

Thornfeldt CR et al 2006. Treatment of Muco-Cutaneous Disorders through Reversing Chronic Inflammation and Barrier Disruption. US patent AI.

Vayalil PK 2002. Antioxidant and antimutagenic properties of aqueous extract of date fruit (Phoenix dactylifera L. Arecaceae). J Agric Food Chem. 50; 610-617.

Pine Aleppo and Pine Turkish

Adams F 1844/1846/1847, 3.78, 663, 665. The 7 Books of Paulus Aegineta. Translated from the Greek. London: Sydenham Society. Digital text, Bibliothèque Inter-universitaire de Medicine et d'Odontologie, Paris. http://web2.bium.univ-paris5.fr.

Arnold-Apostolides 1985. Contribution à la connaissance ethnobotanique et médicinale de la flore de Chypre. Ph.D. thesis, Faculté de sciences pharmacologiques et biologiques, Université René Descartes de Paris, Luxembourg.

Berendes J. 1902. Des Pendanius Dioscorides aus Anazarbos Arzneimittellehre in fünf Büchern. Stuttgart: Ferdinand Enke; Digital edition, Heilpflanzen-Welt, Bibliothek. Multi MED vision GbR Berliner Medizinredaktion, Medizin und Medien. Available at: http://buecher.heilpflanzen-welt.de/Dioskurides-Arzneimittellehre/

Cretu E et al 2013. In vitro study on the antioxidant activity of a polyphenol-rich extract from Pinus brutia bark and its fractions.

Dioscorides De Materia Medica 1.91 and 1.93. Trans TA Osbaldeston and RPA Wood. Ibidis Press 2000.

Digrak M et al 1999. Anti-microbial activities of several parts of Pinus brutia, Juniperus oxycedrus, Abies cilicia, Cedrus libani and Pinus nigra. Phytother Res 13 (7), 584-587.

Fernández MA et al 2001. Anti-inflammatory activity of abietic acid, a diterpene isolated from *Pimenta racemosa* var. *grissea*. J. Pharm. Pharmacol. 53, 867–87210.1211/0022357011776027.

Gülçin 2003 et al Antioxidant and analgesic activities of turpentine of *Pinus nigra* Arn. subsp. *pallsiana* (Lamb.) Holmboe. J. Ethnopharmacol. 86, 51–5810.1016/S0378-8741(03)00036-9.

Hadjikyriakou GN 2007. Aromatika kai artymatika fyta stin Kypro. Lefkosia (Nicosia): Politistiko Idryma Trapesis Kyprou.

Lentini A. 2004. Fragrant substances and therapeutic compounds, in Pyrgos-Mavroraki, Advanced Technology in Bronze Age Cyprus, ed. Belgiorno MR. Nicosia: Archaeological Museum; 45–47.

Satil F and Selvi S 2011. Ethnic uses of pine resin production from *Pinus brutia* by native people on the Kazdağ Mountain (Mt. Ida) in Western Turkey. J Food, Agric Envir, 9 (3&4): 1059-1063.

Süntar I et al 2012. Appraisal on the wound healing and anti-inflammatory activities of the essential oils obtained from the cones and needles of Pinus species by in vivo and in vitro experimental models. J Ethnopharmacol 139 (2) 533-540.

Ulukanli Z et al 2014. Chemical composition, anti-microbial and antioxidant activities of Mediterranean Pinus brutia and Pinus pinea resin essential oils.

Yeşilada E et al 1995. Traditional medicine in Turkey. V. Folk medicine in the inner Taurus Mountains. J Ethnopharmacol 46 (3):133-152.

Pine Corsican and Pine stone
Antoninus Liberalis. The Metamorphoses. trans Francis Celoria.

Routledge 1992.

Amr, A 2011. Hypolipidemic and hypocholesteremic effect of pine nuts in rats fed high fat, cholesterol-diet. World Applied Sciences Journal 15 (12): 1667-1677.

Lucian works. Trans AM Harmon, K Kilburn and MD Macleod. Loeb Classical Library, 1913–1967.

Yang R et al 2017. Identification of novel peptides from 3 to 10 kDa pine nut (*Pinus koraiensis*) meal protein, with an exploration of the relationship between their antioxidant activities and secondary structure. Food Chemistry 219; 311-320.

Megre VN 1996. Anastasia. Zveniaschie Kedry Rossii. St. Petersburg: Dilya. 224 p.

Pomegranate tree

Adams LS et al 2006. Pomegranate juice, total pomegranate ellagitannins and punicalagin suppress inflammatory cell signalling in colon cancer cells. J Agric Food Chem. 54; 980-5.

Albrecht M et al 2004. Pomegranate extracts potently suppress proliferation, xenograft growth, and invasion of human prostate cancer cell. J Med Food 7; 274-83.

Al-Zoreky NS 2009. Anti-microbial activity of pomegranate (Punica granatum L.) fruit peels. Int J food Microbiol 134 (3); 244-248.

Apollodorus The library iii. 5. 1. Trans JG Frazer 1963-1967. Loeb Classical library Cambridge MA, Harvard Uni Press.

Campbell Thompson R 1949. Dictionary of Assyrian Botany [DAB] (London: British Academy. 315, 11, and Ebeling, KAR, 194, iv, 18.

Gil MO et al 2000. Antioxidant activity of pomegranate juice and its relationship with phenolic compositions and processing. J Agric Food Chem 48; 4581-9.

Ed Navindra Seeram, Risa Schulman and David Heber. Taylor and Francis.

Homeric Hymns. trans Peter Green 2015 Univ of California Press.

Jacobsen T 1976. The Treasures of Darkness: A History of Mesopotamian Religion. New Haven, CT: Yale University Press. 16, 25–47.

Khan N et al 2007. Pomegranate fruit extract inhibits pro-survival pathways in human A549 lung carcinoma cells and tumour growth in athymic nude mice. Carcinogenesis. 28: 163-73.

Mehta R and Lansky EP 2004. Breast cancer chemo-preventive properties of pomegranate (Punica granatum) fruit extracts in a mouse mammary organ culture. Eur J Cancer Prev. 13;345-8.

Mirmiran P et al 2010. Effect of pomegranate seed oil on hyperlipidaemic subjects; A double-blind-controlled clinical trial. Br J Nutri 104; 402-6.

Newman RA et al 2007. Pomegranate: the most medicinal fruit. Laguna Beach, California: Basic Health Publications - A wealth of Phytochemicals p120.

Oudhia P, Research Note, in http:botanical.com/site/column_poudhis/77_ gyn.html

Pacheco-Palencia LA et al 2008. Protective effects of standardised pomegranate (Punica granatum L.) polyphenolic extract in ultraviolet-irradiated human skin fibroblasts. J Agric Food Chem. 56; 8434-41.

Prakash AO 1986. Potentialities of some indigeneous plants for anti-fertility activity," Internat J Crude Drug Res 24: 21, 23 [19–24].

Rettig MB et al 2008. Pomegranate extract inhibits androgen-independent prostate cancer growth through a nuclear factor-kappa B-dependent mechanism. Mol Cancer Ther. 7; 2662-71.

Seeram NP 2006 et al, eds., Pomegranates: Ancient Roots to Modern Medicine. Boca Raton, FL: CRC Taylor & Francis

Press.

Stone D 2017. A global history. The Edible series. Reaction Books Ltd. London.

Strawberry tree Grecian

Afrin S et al 2017. Strawberry-tree honey induces growth inhibition of human colon cancer cells and increases ROS generation: A comparison with Manuka honey. Int. J. Mol. Sci. 2017, 18(3), 613.

Fortalezas S et al 2010. Antioxidant properties and neuroprotective capacity of strawberry tree fruit (Arbutus unedo). Nutrients 2010, 2(2), 214-229.

Jurica K et al 2017. Arbutin and its metabolite hydroquinone as the main factors in the anti-microbial effect of strawberry tree (Arbutus unedo L.) leaves. J Herbal Med 8: 17-23.

Jurica K et al 2018. In vitro safety assessment of the strawberry tree (Arbutus unedo L.) water leaf extract and arbutin in human peripheral blood lymphocytes. Cytotechnol 70: 1261-1278.

Oliveira I 2009. Scavenging capacity of strawberry tree (Arbutus unedo L.) leaves on free radicals. Food and Chemical Toxicology 47 (7): 1507-1511.

Orak HH et al 2011. Evaluation of antioxidant and anti-microbial potential of strawberry tree (Arbutus Unedo L.) leaf. Food Sci Biotechnol 20: 1249.

Tavares L et al 2010. Antioxidant and antiproliferative properties of strawberry tree tissues. J Berry Res 1 (1): 3-12.

Willow white

Apollonius Rhodius Argonautica. Trans WH Race 2008. Loeb Classical Library 1. Cambridge MA and London: Harvard University Press.

Graves R 1948. The White Goddess. Faber and Faber.

Hippocrates. Corpus Hippocraticum. Henderson J ed. Trans

Loeb Vols 1-4 1923–1931 Heinemann London. Loeb Vols 5-10 1988 - 2012 Harvard Uni Press.

Homer Hymn to Demeter. Trans Foley HP 1993. Princeton University Press (NJ)

Jack DB 1997. One hundred years of aspirin. Lancet, 350: 437-439.

Newall C, Anderson I, Phillipson JD 1996. Herbal Medicines - A guide for health-care professionals. Pharmaceutical Press 1996.

Riddle JM 1999. Historical data as an aid in pharmaceutical prospecting and drug safety determination. J. Alt. Complement Med., 5 (2); 195-201.

Stone E 1763. An account of the success of the bark of the willow in the cure of agues. Philos. Trans., 53: 195.

Sutcliffe J and Dunn N 1992. A History of Medicine. Barnes and Noble, NY

Wells, JCD 2003. Poppy juice and willow bark: Advances in their use for the 21st Century. The Pain Web for Health Professionals. http://www.thepainweb.com

Illustration Credits

Oak Valonia *Quercus ithaburensis macrolepis*
The British Library - page 283 of &#039
Notes of a military reconnaissance from Port Leavenworth in Missouri to San Diego,
in California, including parts of the Arkansas, del Norte and Gila Rivers
No restrictions, wiki commons

Almond *Prunus amygdalus or dulcis*

François Rozier - http://bibdigital.rjb.csic.es/ing/Libro.php?Libro=5979
Public Domain, wiki commons

Apple tree *Malus domestica*

https://wellcomeimages.org/indexplus/image/V0043140.html
Wellcome Collection gallery (2018-03-23): wiki commons

Ash Manna Ash *Fraxinus ornus*

From wiki commons

Chaste tree *Vitex agnus castus*

From wiki commons

Cherry tree Cornelian *Cornus mas*

Loudon   JC   -   https://www.flickr.com/photos/biodivlibrary/
6918267252
Public Domain, wiki commons

Fig tree *Ficus carica*

The British Library - page 159 of '
Das republikanische Brasilien in Vergangenheit und Gegenwart,
etc.
No restrictions, wiki commons

Frankincense tree *Boswellia carterii*

From wiki commons

Laurel or Bay Sweet *Laurus nobilis*

Meyer, Frederick G. 1917-2006; Mazzeo, Peter M;Voss, Donald
H; National Arboretum (U.S.) https://www.flickr.com/
photos/internetarchivebookimages/20387329658/
No restrictions, wiki commons

Lime or linden, Large-leafed *Tilia platyphyllos*

Dr. Karl Rothe, Ferdinand Frank, Josef Steigl - Naturgeschichte
für Bürgerschulen. Vienna 1895, Verlag von A. Pichler &
#039;s Witwe & Sohn.,

Public Domain, wiki commons

Lotus tree or Date plum *Diospyrus lotus*
From wiki commons

Mulberry black *Morus nigra*
Edward Step - From the Biodiversity Heritage Library
biodiversitylibrary.org/item/67168
Public Domain, wiki commons

Myrrh tree *Commiphora myrrha*
From wiki commons

Myrtle *Myrtus communis*
Penzig, O. https://www.flickr.com/photos/biodivlibrary/62444
    57740, Public Domain
https://commons.wikimedia.org/w/index.php?curid=42760917

Olive tree *Olea europaea*
From wiki commons

Palm Date *Phoenix dactylifera*
H.M. Dixon - Flickr: Date Palm Page 785
Public Domain, wiki commons

Pine Aleppo and Pine Turkish *Pinus halepensis* and *Pinus brutia*
Zeynel Cebeci CC BY-SA 4.0 https://commons.wikimedia.
    org/w/index.php?curid=37085817

Pine Corsican and Pine stone *Pinus nigra laricio* and *Pinus pinea*

Bauer, Ferdinand; Don, David; Lambert, Aylmer Bourke
https://www.flickr.com/photos/biodivlibrary/7797271162
Public Domain, wiki commons

Pomegranate tree *Punica granatum*
From wiki commons

Strawberry tree Grecian *Arbutus andrachne* and *Arbutus unedo*
Adamovic, Lujo (Lujo V.), b. 1869 - https://www.flickr.com/photos/
internetarchivebookimages/20753399539/Source book page:
https://archive.org/stream/diepflanzenweltd00adam/#page/
n232/mode/1up
No restrictions, wiki commons

Willow white *Salix alba*
https://commons.wikimedia.org/w/index.php?curid=2358667

The Pants and Flowers of Ancient Greek Myth
Athenaeus The Learned Banquet (Deipnosophistai). Trans CD
Yonge 1819. Henry Bohn London.
Bauman H 1982. The Greek plant world in myth, art and
literature. 1993 Timber Press.
Dioscorides De Materia Medica. Trans TA Osbaldeston and RPA
Wood. Ibidis Press 2000.
Herodotus Histories. Trans by George Rawlinson, with the
notes abridged by AJ Grant,
British Library, Historical Print Editions 2011.
Hesiod 730-700 BCE. Theogony. Trans HG Evelyn-White 2017
by Createspace Independent Publishing Platform.
Homer Odyssey trans P Green 2015. Uni California Press.
Homer Iliad trans P Green 2019 Uni California Press.
Pausanias Guide to Greece. Trans Jones WHS and Ormerod HA
Loeb Classical Library. Cambridge, MA, Harvard Uni Press;

London, Heinemann 1918.

Pliny Natural History. Trans H Rackham vols 1-5, 9 WHS Jones vols 6-8 and DE Eichholz vol 10. London: Heinemann; Cambridge, Mass: Harvard University Press, 1938-1963.

Theocritus Idylls. Trans Trevelyan RC. Osmania Uni Library.

Theophrastus. Historia Plantarum. Trans Sir Arthur Hort 1916 Loeb Classical Library.

Xenophon Anabasis. Trans by HG Dakyns 2013.

Artemisia, the "Mother Herb"

Arnold WN 1988. Vincent van Gogh and the Thujone Connection," J Am Med Ass 260/20: 3042-44.

BBC News, February 8, 2003: http//newsvote.bbc.co.uk/mpapps/ pagetools/print/

news. bbc.co.uk/2.html (accessed 8/25/08).

Bently P ed. 1995. Dictionary of World Myth. New York: Facts on File 25.

Caner, Ayşe et al 2008. Comparison of the Effects of *Artemisia vulgaris* and *Artemisia absinthium* growing in Western Anatolia against Trichinellosis (*Trichinella spiralis*) in Rats," Experimental Parasitology 1119/1: 173–179.

Celsus, De medicina, for *abrotonum* (southernwood) 4. 8.3–4 (1: 386 Spencer ed.).

Chiassonetal H 2001. Acaricidal properties of *Artemisia absinthium* and *Tanacetum vulgare* (Asteraceae) essential oils obtained by 3 methods of extraction," Journal of Economic Entomology 94/1: 167–171.

Dioscorides, De materia medica, 3. 113. Beck, trans. 233.

Dioscorides, De materia medica, 1. 104. 1. 4, Max Wellmann ed., Berlin, 1958 repr., vol. 1, p. 96.

Duplais P 1871. A Treatise on the manufacture and distillation of alcoholic liquors. M. McKennie trans from French. Philadelphia, PA: Baird, 1871. 244.

EDrugDigest: http://www.drugdigest.org/DD/DVH/HerbsWh

o/0,3923,4064 | Wormwood,00.html.

Galen. De simpl. med. temp. ac fac, 6. 1 (Kühn ed., 11: 798–807, 839–840; *De methodo medendi,* 11. 16 (expel poisons; K. 10: 789–790); 8. 5 (K. 10: 572); *De sanitate tuenda,* 6. 7 (K. 6: 428); *De alimentorum facultatibus.* 3. 32 (K. 6: 731); *De antidotis.* 2.7 (K. 14: 140).

Galen, De simpl. med. temp. ac fac, 6.1 (11: 804).

Hemingway E 1940. For whom the bell tolls. New York: Charles Scribner's. 50.

Mascetti MD 1996. Artemis: Goddess of the hunt and moon. San Francisco: Chronicle Books, 1996. 16–18.

Martin H M 1903. "Artemis,"in ABD, 1:464–465; see also Wernicke, "Artemis," in Paulys Real-encyclopädie der classischen Altertumswissenschaft. Stuttgart: Metzler, 2/1: 1335–1440.

Rekand T and Sulg I 2003. Absint og den kunstneriske kreativitet. Tidsskrift for

den Norske laegeforening tidsskrift for praktish medicinem ny reakke, 123/1. 70 –73.

Riddle J 1997. Eve's Herbs: A History of Contraception and Abortion in the West. Cambridge, MA: Harvard University Press. 47–48, 56, 83, 86, 89–92, 98, 103–104, 114, 122–124, 137, 154, 161.

Pliny Natural History, 25. 34. 73

Pseudo-Apuleius's Herbarius, 12. 2. Ernest Howald and Henry Sigerist, eds. 45.

Smith PEM 2006. Absinthe Attacks. Neurology and Art 6: 376–381;

Soranus, Gynecology, Oswei Temkin, trans. Baltimore: Johns Hopkins University Press, 1956, 1. 64. 66–67.

Wright, CW 2002. *Artemisia.* London and New York: Taylor and Francis, ix; Hongwe Yu and Shouming Zhong, "*Artemisia species* in Traditional Chinese Medicine and the Discovery of Artemisinin," in Artemisia, 156.

Zheng T and Tang 1988. p. 300 (with other references); Stephen O. Duke, Rex.

N. Paul, and Lee S. Mark, "Terpenoids from the genus *Artemisia* as Potential Pesticides," in Biologically Active Natural Products. Symposium. American Chemical Society 194 (1988/3802): 318–334.

Asparagus

Alok S 2013 Plant profile, phytochemistry and pharmacology of Asparagus racemosus (Shatavari): A review. Asian Pac J Trop Dis. 3 (3): 242-251.

Bhatnagar M and Sisodia SS 2006. Anti-secretory and anti-ulcer activity of Asparagus racemosus Willd. Against indomethacin plus pyloric ligation-induced gastric ulcer in rats. J Herb Pharmacother. 6 (1): 13-20.

De B et al 1997. Effect of some Sitavirya drugs on gastric secretion and ulceration. Indian J Exp Biol. 35: 1084-1087.

Food as Medicine: Asparagus. Asparagus officinalis Asparagaceae Editor's Note Each Month 2016 HerbalEGram February 2016 13 (2).

Gautam M et al 2009. Immunomodulatory activity of Asparagus racemosus on systemic Th1/Th2 immunity: implications for immune adjuvant potential. J Ethno Pharmacol. 121 (2): 241-247.

Iqbal M et al 2017. Review on therapeutic and Pharmaceutically Important Medicinal Plant Asparagus officinalis. J Plant Biochem and Physiol. 5:1 DOI: 10.4172/2329-9029. 1000180.

Joglekar GV et al 1967. Galactogogue effect of Asparagus racemosus. Indian Med J. 61: 165.

Mandal et al 2000. Antitussive effect of Asparagus racemosus root against sulfur dioxide-induced cough in mice. Fitoterapia 71 (6): 686.

Mandal et al 2000. Evaluation of anti-bacterial activity of Asparagus racemosus Willd. root. Phytother Res. 14 (2): 118-

119.

Nishimura M et al 2013. Improvement of Blood Pressure, Glucose Metabolism, and Lipid Profile by the Intake of Powdered Asparagus (Lú Sǔn) Bottom-stems and Cladophylls. J Trad Comp Med. 3 (4); 250-255.

Sanae M, Yasuo A 2013. Green asparagus (Asparagus officinalis) prevented hypertension by an inhibitory effect on angiotensin-converting enzyme activity in the kidney of spontaneously hypertensive rats. J Agric Food Chem: 61 (23): 5520-5525.

Sharma PC et al 2000. Data based on medicinal plants used in Ayurveda. Delhi: Documentation and publication division: Central council for research in Ayurveda and Sidha 1: 418-430.

Thakur S and Sharma DR 2015. Review on medicinal plant: *Asparagus adscendens* Roxb. Int J Pharma Sci Health Care 5: 82-97.

Zhu X et al 2010. Hypolipidaeic and hepatoprotective effects of ethanol and aqueous extracts from Asparagus officinalis L. by-products in mice fed a high-fat diet. J Sci Food Agric. 90 (7): 1129-1135.

Celery and Parsley

Anand NK et al 1981. Coumarins from *Apium petroselinum* seeds. Natl Acad sci Lett; 4: 249-251.

Alireza Y et al 2012. Immunomodulatory effect of parsley (*Petroselimum crispum*) essential oil on immune cells: Mitogen-activated splenocytes and peritoneal macrophages, Immunopharmacolgy and Immunotoxicol, Transplant Res Center, Shiraz, Iran. 34 (2): 303-308.

Apollodorus The library. Trans JG Frazer 1963-1967. Loeb Classical library Cambridge MA, Harvard Uni Press.

Baytop T 1984. Therapy with medicinal plants in turkey (Past and present), Istanbul University Yayinlari, Turkey p 3255.

Bolkent S et al 2004. Effects of Parsley (*Petroselinum crispum*) on the liver of diabetic rats. A morphological and biochemical study. Phytother Res 18: 996-999.

Chaves DS et al 2011. Phenolic chemical composition of *Petroselinum crispum* extract and its effect on haemostasis. Nat Prod Commun. 6 (7): 961-964.

Fraga CG et al 1987. Flavonoids as antioxidants evaluated by *in vitro* and *in situ* liver chemiluminescence. Bioch Pharmacol 36: 717-720.

Hempel J et al 1999. Flavonols and flavones of parsley cell suspension culture change the anti oxidative capacity of plasma in rats. Nahrun. 43: 201-204.

Janssen K et al 1998. Effects of the flavonoids quercetin and apigenin on homeostasis in healthy volunteers: results from an *in vitro* and a dietary supplement study. Am J Clin Nutr. 67: 255-262.

Jeong YJ et al 2007. Attenuation of monocyte adhesion and oxidised LDL uptake in luteolin-treated human endothelial cells exposed to oxidised LDL. Br J Nurt. 97: 447-457.

Kitagawa I et al 1976. Structures of 3 soybean saponins: soyssaponin II, and soyasaponin III. Chem Pharm Bull. 24: 121-129.

Lee SJ et al 1993. Anti-inflammatory activity of naturally occurring flavone and flavonoids glycosides. Archives of Pharmacol Res. 16: 25-28.

Mahmood M 2014. Critique of medicinal conspicuousness of Parsley *(Petroselinum crispum)*: A culinary herb of Mediterranean region. Pakistan journal of pharmaceutical sciences. November.

Manthey JA et al 2002. Anti-proliferative activities of citrus flavonoids against 6 human cancer cell lines. J Aric Food chef. 50: 5837-5843.

Marczal G et al 1997. Phenolether components of diuretic effect in parsley I. Acta Agron Acad. Sci Hung., 26: 7-13.

Nielsen et al 1999. Effect of parsley intake on urinary apigenin excretion, blood antioxidant enzymes and biomarkers for oxidative stress in human subjects. Br J Nutr 81: 447-455.

Ozsoy et al 2006. Effects of parsley (*Petroselinum crispum*) extract versus glibornuride on the liver of streptozotocin-induced diabetic rats. J. Ethnopharmacol. 104 (1-2): 175-181.

Ozturk et al 1991. Hepatoprotective (antihepatotoxic) plants in turkey. Proceedings of the 9th Symposium of Plant Drugs. Eskisehir Turkey, 40-50.

Pino JA et al 1996. Herb oil of parsley (*Petroselinum crispum* Mill.) from Cuba. J Essent Oil Res., 9: 241-242.

Ueda H et al 2004. A hydroxyl group of flavonoids affects oral anti-inflammatory activity and inhibition of systemic tumour necrosis factor-alpha production. Biosci. Biotechnol. Biochem. 68: 119-125.

Vora S R et al 2009. Protective effects of *Petroselinum crispum* (Mill) Nyman ex AW Hill leaf extract on D-galactose-induced oxidative stress in mouse brain. Indian J Exp Biol 47 (05): 338-342.

Wong PYY and Kitts DD 2006. Studies on the dual antioxidant and anti-bacterial properties of parsley (*Petroselinum crispum*) and cilantro (*Foriandum sativum*) extracts. Food Chem, 97: 505-515.

Ziyyat A et al 1997. Phytotherapy of hypertension and diabetes in oriental Morocco. J Ethnopharmacol. 58: 45-54.

Crocus saffron

Abe K and Saito H 2000. Effects of saffron extract and its constituent crocin on learning behaviour and long-term potentiation. Phytother Res. 14 (3): 1499-52.

Ahmad AS et al 2005. Neuro-protection by crocetin in a hemi-parkinsonian rat model. Pharmacol Biochem behave 81 (4): 805-13.

Akhondzadeh S et al 2005. Crocus sativus L in the treatment

of mild to moderate depression: a double-blind, randomised
and placebo controlled trial. Phytother Res 19 (2): 148-151.

Assimopoulou AN et al 2005. Radical scavenging activity of
Crocus sativus L extract and its bioactive constituents.
Phytother Res. 19 (11): 997-1000.

Bhargavak V 2011. Medicinal uses and pharmacological
properties of Crocus sativus Linn (Saffron). Int J Pharm and
Parmaceut Sci 3 (3).

Boskabody MH 2006. Relaxant effect of Crocus sativus (saffron)
on guinea-pig tracheal chains and its possible mechanisms. J
Pharm Pharmacol. 58 (10): 1385-90.

Chatterjee S et al 2005. Emollient and antipruritic effect of itch
cream in dermatological disorders: A randomised controlled
trial. Res Lett: 37 (4): 253-254.

Homeric Hymns. trans Peter Green 2015 Univ of California
Press.

Hosseinzadeh H and Talebzadeh F 2005. Anticonvulsant
evaluation of safranal and crocin from Crocus sativus in
mice. Fitoterapia 76: 722-724.

Noorbala AA et al 2005. Hydro-alcoholic extract of Crocus
sativus L versus fluoxetine in the treatment of mild to
moderate depression: a double-blind, randomised pilot trial.
J Ethnopharmacol 97 (2): 281-284.

Ovid The Metamorphoses. Trans AS Kline 2000. Pan American.

Papandreou MA et al 2006. Inhibitory activity on amyloid-beta
aggregation and antioxidant properties of Crocus sativus
stigmas extract and its crocin constituents. J Agric Food
Chem; 54 (23): 8762-8.

Rios JL et al 1996. An update review of saffron and its active
constituents. Phytother Res 10 (3): 189-193.

Souret FF and Weathers P 2000. Cultivation, in vitro culture,
secondary metabolite production and phytopharmacognosy
of saffron (Crocus sativus L.) J Herbs, Spices Med Plants. 6
(4): 99-116.

Verma SK and Bordia A 1998. Antioxidant property of saffron in man. Indian J Med Sci 52 (5): 205-207.

Willburn AJ et al 2004. The natural treatment of hypertension. J Clin Hypertens 6 (5): 242-248.

Xi L et al 2006. Beneficial impact of crocetin, a carotenoid from saffron, on insulin sensitivity in fructose-fed rats. J Nutr Biochem 18 (1): 64-72.

Xuan B et al 1999. Effects of crocin analogues on ocular blood flow and retinal function. J Ocul Pharmacol there. 15 (2): 143-52.

Dittany

Aristotle. Historia Animalia 9.16.1. History of Animals. Trans Michael Scot. E-Book (Pdf) 2020.

Baumann H 1996. Greek wild flowers and plant lore in ancient Greece. The Herbert Press Ltd, London.

Bazaios K 1982. 100 herbs for 1000 therapies. Athens.

Berendes J 1902. Des Pedanios Diokurides aus Anazarbos Arzeinmittellhre in fünf Büchern. Verlag von Enke, Stuttgart; 284-285.

Chatzopoulou A 1985. Depsides and other polar constituents from Origanum dictamnus L. and there in vitro anti-microbial activity in clinical strains. J Agric Food Chem. 58 (10): 6064-6068.

Couladis et al 2003. Screening of some Greek aromatic plants for antioxidant activity. Phytother Res 17 (2): 194-195.

Diapoulis HA 1980. Prehistoric Plants of the islands of the Aegean Sea, Sea Daffodils (Pancratium maritimus), Thera and the Aegean World II, London: 129-139.

Dioscorides De Materia Medica. Fifth book. 3.37. Trans TA Osbaldeston and RPA Wood. Ibidis Press 2000.

EMA/HMPC, 2013. Final assessment report on Origanum dictamnus L herba (200431/2012). European Medicines Agency/Committee on Herbal Medicinal Products, London.

Exarchou et al 2013. 4 new depsides in Origanum dictamnus methanol extract. Phytochem Lett 6: 46-52.

Gennadios P 1914. Lexicon Phytologicon. Athens.

Hippocrates. Corpus Hippocraticum. Henderson J ed. Trans Loeb Vols 1-4 1923–1931 Heinemann London. Loeb Vols 5-10 1988 - 2012 Harvard Uni Press.

Homer. Iliad 11.843-847. trans P Green 2019 Uni California Press.

Hunt P 2005. Aeneid XII. 383-440 as inspiration for ancient art: the Roman surgeon.

Karanika MS et al 2001. Effect of aqueous extracts of some plants of Lamiaceae family on the growth of Yarrowia lipolytica. Int J food Microbiol 64 (1-2): 175-181.

Komaitis ME et al 1988. The lipid composition of fresh Origanum dictamnus leaves. Food Chem 27 (1): 25-32.

Liolios CC et al 2010 Dittany of Crete: a botanical and ethnopharmacological review. J Ethnopharmacol.

Plimakis AG 1997. Dictamnus the miraculous herb of Crete. Hania, Greece. (in Greek)

Plutarch. 2nd century AD.

Revonthe-Moraiti K et al 1985. Identification and quantitative determination of the lipids of dried Origanum dictamnus leaves. Food Chem 16: 15-24.

Sivropoulou A et al 1996. Anti-microbial and cytotoxic activities of Origanum essential oils. J Aric Food Chem 44 (5) 1202-1205.

Skoula M and Kamenopoulos S 1997. Origanum dictamnus L and Origanum vulgare L subs hirtum: traditional uses and production in Greece. In: Padulosi S (ed). Proceedings of the IPGRI International Workshop on Oregano 8-12 May 1996. CIHEAM, Valenzano, Bari, Italy: 26-32.

Scrubs B 1979. Origanum dictamnus L, a Greek native plant. J Ethnopharmacol 1 (4): 411-415.

Thanos CA 1994. Aristotle and Theophrastus on plant-animal

interaction. M Arianoutsou, RH Goves Eds. Plant-Animal interactions in Mediterranean-type ecosystems, Kluwer Academic Publishers, Dordrecht, The Netherlands: 3-11.

Theophrastus. Historia Plantarum. Trans Sir Arthur Hort 1916 Loeb Classical Library.

Virgil's Aeneid 1st century BCE. Book XII. 411-415. Loeb translation.

Elecampane

Theophrastus Enquiry into Plants 9.9.2 Trans Hort AF 1916. Loeb Classical Library.

Garlic

Aristophanes. The complete plays. Trans Paul Roche. New American Library 2005.

Dioscorides De Materia Medica. 3.37. Trans TA Osbaldeston and RPA Wood. Ibidis Press 2000.

Herodotus Histories. Trans by George Rawlinson. with the notes abridged by AJ Grant, British Library, Historical Print Editions 2011.

Hippocrates. Corpus Hippocraticum. Henderson J ed. Trans Loeb Vols 1-4 1923–1931 Heinemann London. Loeb Vols 5-10 1988 - 2012 Harvard Uni Press.

Petrovska BB 2010. Extracts from the history and medical properties of garlic. Pharmacogn Rev. Jan-Jun; 4(7): 106–110.

Gentian

Ahmadi F et al 2010. Chemical composition, *in vitro* antimicrobial, anti-fungal and antioxidant activities of the essential oil and methanolic extract of *Hymenocrater longiflorus* Benth., of Iran. Food Chem Toxicol. 48: 1137-1144.

Chen FP. 2008. Frequency and pattern of Chinese herbal medicine prescriptions for chronic hepatitis in Taiwan. J Ethnopharmacol: 117 (1): 84-91.

Chen YJ et al 2016. Complementary therapies in medicine 26, 21-27.

Dioscorides De Materia Medica. 3.3 Trans TA Osbaldeston and RPA Wood. Ibidis Press 2000.

Kumarasamy Y et al 2003. Bioactivity of gentiopicroside from the aerial parts of Centaurium erythraea. Fitoterapia, 74: 151–154.

Mihailovitc V et al 2011. Studies on the anti-microbial activity and chemical composition of the essential oils and alcoholic extracts of Gentiana asclepiadea L. J Med Plants Res 5 (7): 1164-1174.

Mihailovitc V et al 2013. Chemical composition, antioxidant and anti-genotoxic activities of different fractions of Gentiana asclepiadea L. roots extract. Excli J 2013; 12: 807-823.

Mihailovitc V et al 2013. Hepatoprotective effects of Gentiana asclepiadea L extracts against carbon tetrachloride induced liver injury in rats. Food Toxicol. 52: 83-90.

Mirzaee F et al 2017. Medicinal, biological and phytochemical properties of Gentiana species. J Trad and Compl Med 7 (4); 400-408.

Nayebi E et al Appetizing effect of Gentiana olivieri extract in children with anorexia. J Mazandaran Univ Med Sci. 2016 (133): 58-66.

Pliny Natural History. Trans H Rackham vols 1-5, 9.

DE Suciu M et al 2012. Preliminary results on study of the hepatoprotective and anti-microbial effects of *Gentiana ascepiadea* ethanol extract. Annals of RSCB; XVII, 2.

Zajac A and Pindel A 2011. Review of the willow gentian, Gentiana asclepiadea L Biodiversity 12.

Zhao ZL 2010. Identification of medicinal plants used as Tibetan traditional medicine jie-ji. J Ethnopharmacol 2010; 132 (1): 122-126.

Grape vine

Akaberi M and Hosseinzadeh H 2016. Grapes (*Vitis vinifera*) as a Potential Candidate for the therapy of the metabolic syndrome. Phytother Res 30 (4): 540-556.

Athenaeus. Deipnosophistai ("The Gastronomers") Trans C.D. Yonge 1854.

Homer Illiad. Trans P Green 2015. Uni California Press.

Baur et al 2006. Resveratrol improves health and survival of mice on a high-calorie diet. Nature, 444: 337-342.

Brasnyó et al 2011 Resveratrol improves insulin sensitivity, reduces oxidative stress and activates the Akt pathway in type 2 diabetic patients. Br. J. Nutr., 106 (2011), pp. 383-389.

Cals-Grieson MM 2003. Plant extract of the species *Vitis vinifera* as NO-synthase inhibitor and uses. US Patent App. 10/258,814, 2003.

Elsherbini SH 1999. Squalene is an anti-viral compound for treating hepatitis C virus carriers. U. S. Patent, 5858389. (Port Reading, NJ).

Gruber et al 2007. Evidence for a trade-off between survival and fitness caused by resveratrol treatment of Caenorhabditis elegans. Ann. N Y Acad. Sci., 1100: 530-542.

Hemmati AA et al 2011. Topical grape (*Vitis vinifera*) seed extract promotes repair of full thickness wound in rabbit. Internat Wound J 8 (5): 514-520.

Isler-Kerényi C and Watson W. 2007. Dionysos in Archaic Greece: An understanding through images. Leiden; Boston: Brill.

Jayaprakasha GK 2003. Anti-bacterial and antioxidant activities of grape (Vitis vinifera) seed extracts. Food Research International. 36 (2): 117-122.

Jun Park S et al 2012. Resveratrol Ameliorates aging-related metabolic phenotypes by inhibiting cAMP phosphodiesterases. Cell 148 (3): 421-433.

Lagouge M et al 2006. Resveratrol improves mitochondrial function and protects against metabolic disease by activating SIRT1 and PGC-1alpha. Cell, 127: 1109-1122.

Naseri G et al 2006. Spasmolytic effect of Vitis vinifera leaf extract on rat colon. DARU Journal of Pharmaceutical Sciences. 14 (4): 203-207.

Nonnus Dionysiaca 11.185 Trans Rouse. Cambridge, Mass., Harvard University Press, 1955-1956.

Shivananda Nayak B 2010. Wound-healing activity of the skin of the common grape (Vitis vinifera) variant, cabernet sauvignon. Phytother Res 24 (8): 1151-1157.

Thorsten M et al 2009. Residues of grape (*Vitis vinifera* L.) seed oil production as a valuable source of phenolic antioxidants. Food Chem., 112 (3): 551–559.

Iris

Basser K et al 2011. Composition of volatiles from 3 Iris species of Turkey. J Essent Oil Res. 23 (4): 66-71.

Bonfils JP et al 2001. Cytotoxicity of iridals, triterpenoids from Iris, on human tumour cell lines A2780 and K562. Planta Med 67:79–81.

Cumo C ed 2013. Encyclopedia of cultivated Plants: From Acacia to Zinnia ABC-CLIO, Santa Barbara, California USA 1:532-533.

Hacibekiroglu I, Kolak U (2011) Antioxidant and anticholinesterase constituents from the petroleum ether and chloroform extracts of Iris suaveolens. Phytother Res 25: 522–529.

Huwaitat S et al 2013. Antioxidant and anti-microbial activities of Iris nigricans methanol extracts containing phenolic compounds. European Scient. J 9 (3).

Lim TK 2016. Edible Medicinal and Non-Medicinal Plants: Volume 11 Modified Stems, Roots and Bulbs. Springer Internat Pub AG Switzerland pp 3 and 28.

Mosihuzzman M et al 2013. Studies on a-glucosidase inhibition and anti-glycation potential of Iris loczyi and Iris unguicularis. Life Sci 92:187–192.

Orhan I et al 2003. 2 isoflavones and bioactivity spectrum of crude extracts of Iris germanica rhizomes. Phytother Res 17: 575–577.

Pausanias 9.14.7. Guide to Greece Trans Jones WHS and Omerod HA Loeb Classical Library. Cambridge, MA, Harvard Uni Press; London, Heinemann 1918.

Rahman et al 2003. Isoflavonoid glycosides from the rhizomes of Iris germanica. Helv Chim Acta 86: 3354-3362.

Ramtin M et al 2013. Comparative evaluation of the antibacterial activities of essential oils of Iris pseudacorus and Urtica dioica native to north Iran. J Pure Appl Microbiol 7:1065–1070.

Roger B et al 2012. Characterisation and quantification of flavonoids in Iris germanica L. and Iris pallida Lam. Resinoids from Morocco. Phytochem Anal 23:450–455.

Schutz C, et al 2011. Profiling of isoflavonoids in Iris germanica rhizome extracts by microprobe NMR and HPLC–PDA–MS analysis. Fitoterapia 82:1021–1026.

Wollenweber E et al 2003. Cancer Chemopreventive in vitro activities of isoflavones isolated from Iris germanica. Plants Med. 69: 15-20.

Wuttke W et al 2002. Use of extracts and preparation from iris plants and tectorigenin as medicaments. US Patent 20,040,176,310.

Crisan I 2016. New perspectives on medicinal properties and uses of Iris sp. Hop and Medicinal Plants, Year XXIV no 1-2. [A useful review].

Mallow

Dioscorides De Materia Medica. 3.3 Trans TA Osbaldeston and RPA Wood. Ibidis Press 2000.

Grieves M 1931. A Modern Herbal. Johnathon Cape 1992.

Hyginus, Fabulae 171.

Meadowsweet

Pliny, Hist. Nat. 23.5.9.

Theophrastus. Historia Plantarum. 6.68 Trans Sir Arthur Hort 1916 Loeb Classical Library.

Mistletoe

Marze; 1923. Die mistel in der volkskunde. In K con Tubeuf (ed). Monographic der Mistel. R Oldenburg Verlag, Machen Berlin pp28-37.

Pliny Natural History. Trans H Rackham.

Virgil Aenid 6.205 trans Frederick Ahl 2007.

Peony

Abdel-Aty, AS 2007. Nematicidal effect of *Paeonia Suffruticosa* Constituents. Alexandria Sci. Exchange J. 28, 1.

Aen vii. 769.

Arentz S, et al 2014. Herbal medicine for the management of polycystic ovary syndrome (PCOS) and associated oligo/amenorrhoea and hyperandrogenism; a review of the laboratory evidence for effects with corroborative clinical findings. BMC Complement Altern Med; 14 (1): 511.

Au TK 2001. A comparison of HIV-1 integrate inhibition by aqueous and methanol extracts of Chinese medicinal herbs. Elsevier 68 (14); 1687-1694.

Ding H-Y 2013. Phytochemical and pharmacological studies on Chinese Paeonia species. J Chinese Chem Soc 47 (2); 381-388.

Ding ZJ et al 2017. Interactions between traditional Chinese medicine and anticancer drugs in chemotherapy. World J Tradit Chin Med; 3 (3): 38-45.

Fang L et al 2013. Effects of Chinese medicines for notifying the kidney on DNMT1 protein expression in endometrium of infertile women during implantation period. J Altern Complement Med 19 (4): 353-359.

Fang R-C et al 2012. The traditional Chinese medicine

prescription pattern of endometriosis patients in Taiwan: a population-based study. Evid Based Complement Alternat Med: 591391.

Goto H et al 2011. A Chinese herbal medicine, Tokishakuyakusan, reduces the worsening of impairments and independence after stroke: a 1-year randomised, controlled trial. Evid Based Complement Altern Med; 194046.

Hirai A et al 1983. Kumagai, Studies on the mechanism of anti-aggregatory effect of *Moutan* Cortex Thromb. Res. 31, 29.

Homer Iliad 5. 401. 899. 902

Iwasaki K et al 2004. A randomized, double-blind, placebo-controlled clinical trial of the Chinese herbal medicine "ba wei di huang wan" in the treatment of dementia J Am Geriat Soc.52: 1518-1521.

Jang JB et al 2009. Therapeutic effects of Chiljehyangbuhwan on primary dysmenorrhea: a randomized, double blind, placebo-controlled study. Complement Ther Med. Jun 2009;17(3): 123-130.

Kim KH et al 2016. The effect of dangguijagyag-san on mild cognitive impairment. J Altern Complement Med; 22 (7): 509-514.

Lee SJ et al In vitro anti-viral activity of 1,2,3,4,6-Penta-O-galloyl-beta-D-glucose against Hepatitis B. Virus Biol Pharm Bull 29, 2131.

Lee S-M et al 2008. Protective effects of Paeonia lactiflora pall on hydrogen peroxide-induced apoptosis in PC12 cells. Biosci. Biotechnol. Biochem.,72, 1272–1277.

Liapina LA et al 2000. Phytochemical and biological studies of Paeoniaceae. Akad.

Liu ZL et al 2013. Chinese herbal medicines for hypertriglyceridaemia. Cochrane Database Syst Rev. June 6, 2013;6:CD009560. doi: 10.1002/14651858.CD009560. pub2. Nauk. Ser. Biol./Ross. Akad. Nauk. 2000, 345.

Nikolova P and Ivanovska N 2008. Estimation and immunological properties of flower and root extracts from Paeonia peregrina. J Herbs, Spices and Med Plants 6 (4).

Pliny Nat. Hist. X-XIV, cap. 10.

Salameh F et al 2008. The effectiveness of combined Chinese herbal medicine and acupuncture in the treatment of atopic dermatitis. J Altern Complement Med; 14 (8): 1043-1048.

Soph Oed Tyr 154.

Theophrastus Enquiry into Plants IX, cap. 6. Trans Hort.

Tak J-H et al 2006. Acaricidal activities of paeonol and benzoic acid from *Paeonia suffruticosa* root bark and monoterpenoids against *Tyrophagus putrescentiae* (Acari: Acaridae) Ahn, Pest Manage. Sci; 62, 551.

Tang et al 2009. Clinical and experimental effectiveness of Astragali compound in the treatment of chronic viral hepatitis B. J Internat Med Res; 37: 662-667.

Wang YW and Wang YJ 2007. J. Zhejiang Univ. Tradit. Chin. Med. 31: 240.

Yarnell E 2017. Herbs for rheumatoid arthritis. Altern Complement Ther; 23 (4):149-156.

Yarnell E 2015. Herbal medicine for dysmenorrhea. Altern Complement Ther; 21 (5): 224-228.

Yuan H-N et al 2008. A randomized, crossover comparison of herbal medicine and bromocriptine against risperidone-induced hyperprolactinemia in patients with schizophrenia. J Clin Psychopharmacol. June 2008;28(3): 264-370.

Xu M et al 2009. Adjuvant phytotherapy in the treatment of cervical cancer: a systematic review and meta-analysis. J Altern Complement Med; 15 (12): 1-7.

Xu Y et al 2015. Ren Shen Yangrong Tang for fatigue in cancer survivors: a phase I/II open-label study. J Altern Complement Med; 21(5): 281-287.

St John's wort

Dioscorides De Materia Medica. 3. 50 Trans TA Osbaldeston

and RPA Wood. Ibidis Press 2000.

Valerian

Dioscorides De Materia Medica. 1,7-8. Trans TA Osbaldeston and RPA Wood. Ibidis Press 2000.

Houghton PJ. 1988. The biological activity of Valerian and related plants. J Ethnopharmacol 22 (2):121-42.

Violet sweet

Ovid, Metamorphoses, Volume I: Books 1-8. 650-730. Trans Frank Justus Miller. Revised by G. P. Goold. Loeb Classical Library No 42 Cambridge, Massachusetts: Harvard Uni Press 1916.

Stern J 1970. Pindar's Olympian 6. The American Journal of Philology 91 (3): 332-340. John Hopkins University Press.

Illustration Credits

Wormwood *Artemisia absinthum*
Leonhart Fuchs. New Kreuterbuch
Public Domain, wiki commons

Asparagus *Asparagus acutifolius*
Leonhart Fuchs. New Kreuterbuch
Public Domain, wiki commons

Celery *Apium graveolens*
From wiki commons

Parsley *Petroselinum sativum*
From wiki commons

Crocus saffron *Crocus sativus*
From wiki commons

Dittany *Origanum dictamnus*
From wiki commons

Elecampane *Inula helenium*
From wiki commons

Garlic *Allium sativum*
From wiki commons

Grape vine *Vitis vinifera*
From wiki commons

Iris *I germanica*
From wiki commons

Poisonous Plants in Greek Myth

Becerra Romero D. Las formas habituales de consumir drogas en la Antigüedad a partir de la obra de Porfirio De Abstinecia. Faventia 2006; 28:67-78.

García Gual C. Introducción a la Mitología Griega. Madrid: Alianza; 2007.

Magner LN 1992. A History of Medicine. 2nd ed. New York Marcel Dekker: 31.

Theophrastus; Sir Arthur Hort, translation. Enquiry into plants and minor works on odours and weather signs. London: W. Heinemann, 1916.

Aconite, Monkshood or Wolf's-bane

Ovid, Metamorphoses, Volume I: Books 1-8. Trans Frank Justus Miller. Revised by G. P. Goold. Loeb Classical Library No 42 Cambridge, Massachusetts: Harvard Uni Press 1916.

Bryony black

Dioscorides De Materia Medica. 4.183, 185 Trans TA Osbaldeston and RPA Wood. Ibidis Press 2000.

Bryony white

Dioscorides De Materia Medica. 4.184 Trans TA Osbaldeston
and RPA Wood. Ibidis Press 2000.

Castor oil plant

Dioscorides De Materia Medica. 4.164. Trans TA Osbaldeston
and RPA Wood. Ibidis Press 2000.

Deadly nightshade

Dioscorides De Materia Medica. 4.74. Trans TA Osbaldeston
and RPA Wood. Ibidis Press 2000.

Fennel giant

Appendino G, et al 2001. Oxygenated sesquiterpenoids from a
nonpoisonous Sardinian chemotype of giant fennel (*Ferula communis.*) J Nat Prod. 64:393–395.

Collenette S 1985. An Illustrated Guide to the Flowers of Saudi
Arabia. London: Scorpion Publishing Ltd.

Hesiod. The Homeric Hymns and Homerica. Trans Hugh
G. Evelyn-White. Theogony. Cambridge, MA., Harvard
University Press; London, William Heinemann Ltd. 1914.

Miski M and Mabry TJ 1985. Daucane esters from *Ferula communis* subsp. *communis*. Phytochemistry. 24:1735–1741.

Nguir A et al 2016. Chemical composition and bio-activities of
the essential oil from different organs of *Ferula communis* L.
growing in Tunisia. Medicinal Chemistry Research 25: 515–525

Rubiolo P et al 2006. Analytical Discrimination of Poisonous
and Nonpoisonous Chemotypes of Giant Fennel (*Ferula communis* L.) through their biologically active and volatile
fractions. Agric. Food Chem. 54 (20): 7556-7563.

Hellebore

Apollodorus The Library book 2. 1.1 Trans J G Frazer.

Berendes J 1891. Die Pharmazie bei den anten Kulturvölkern, II Bände, Georg Olms.

Verlagsbuchhandlung, Hildesheim, I, p. 211.

Hippocrates, Potter P (transl.), Harvard University Press, 1988, Vol. V, Diseases I, 72, p. 327.

Lloyd, GET. (Ed. and Intr.,) Hippocratic Writings, Chadwick J and Mann WN (transl.), Penguin Books, London, 1983, Aphorisms, V, 1, p. 222.

Pausanias, Beschreibung Griechenlands, Übersetzt und mit einer Einleitung und Anmerkungen

versehen von Ernst Meyer, II Bände, Artemis Verlag, Stuttgart, 1967, II, p. 533.

Hemlock

Pliny the elder, Natural History. 25.131 and 95. Trans John Bostock.

Henbane white

Dioscorides De materia medica 2.217 and 4.69. Trans TA Osbaldeston and RPA Wood. Ibidis Press 2000.

Graves R 1955. The Greek myths. London: Penguin Books; volumes 1 and 2.

Mandrake

Butler GF. The vegetable neurotics. J Am Med Assoc. 1899;33:1256–8.

Dioscorides, De materia medica, I. 103. 4. 71. 4. 72. Beck trans. Hildesheim, Germany, Olms-Weidmann, 2005. 540 pp.

Goltz D 1974. Studies zur altorien- talischen und Grieschischen Heilkunde: Therapie—Arzneibereitung—Rezeptstruktur. Sudhoffs Archiv, vol. 16 . Wiesbaden: Franz Steiner Verlag, 83.

Hippocrates. *Corpus Hippocraticum.* Henderson J Trans. Loeb Vols 1-4 1923–1931 Heinemann London. Loeb Vols 5-10 1988 – 20.

Homer. Iliad. trans P Green 2019 Uni California Press.

Oppenheim AL 1956. The Assyrian Dictionary of the Oriental Institute of the University of Chicago (Chicago: Oriental Institute and Gluckstadt: J. J. Augustin), 9: 190.

Riddle JM 1997. pp. 57, 142, 183, 185, 189.

Riddle JM 2010. Goddesses, Elixirs, and Witches. Plants and Sexuality throughout Human History. Palgrave Macmillan.

Pliny Natural History. Trans H Rackham. Blackwell's.

Soranus, Gynecology. 3. 45 and 46. 3–4. Trans Temkin.

Stewart A 2009. Wicked Plants. The weed that killed Lincoln's mother and other botanical atrocities. Chapel Hill, NC Algonquin Books: 106.

Theophrastus. Historia Plantarum. Trans Sir Arthur Hort 1916 Loeb Classical Library.

Thompson RC 1926. Assyrian Medical Texts. Proceeding of the Royal Society of Medicine 19. 67, 187–189.

Wilfred G. Lambert, "Devotion: The languages of religion and love," in figurative language in the ancient near east. London: University of London, 1987.

Wilkinson RH 1988. Complete Gods and Goddesses of Ancient Egypt. 186. Thames and Hudson.

Narcissus

Homer Hymn to Demeter Trans. Evelyn-White.

Ovid Metamorphoses 3.441-55. Trans AS Kline 2000. Pan American.

Poppy opium

Dioscorides De Materia Medica. Trans TA Osbaldeston and RPA Wood. Ibidis Press 2000.

Yew

Denny WA 2002. The contribution of synthetic organic chemistry to anticancer drug development. Anticancer Drug Development.

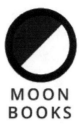

**MOON
BOOKS**

PAGANISM & SHAMANISM

What is Paganism? A religion, a spirituality, an alternative belief
system, nature worship? You can find support for all these defini-
tions (and many more) in dictionaries, encyclopaedias, and text
books of religion, but subscribe to any one and the truth will evade
you. Above all Paganism is a creative pursuit, an encounter with
reality, an exploration of meaning and an expression of the soul.
Druids, Heathens, Wiccans and others, all contribute their insights
and literary riches to the Pagan tradition. Moon Books invites you
to begin or to deepen your own encounter, right here, right now.
If you have enjoyed this book, why not tell other readers by
posting a review on your preferred book site.

Recent bestsellers from Moon Books are:

Journey to the Dark Goddess
How to Return to Your Soul
Jane Meredith
Discover the powerful secrets of the Dark Goddess and
transform your depression, grief and pain into healing
and integration.
Paperback: 978-1-84694-677-6 ebook: 978-1-78099-223-5

Shamanic Reiki
Expanded Ways of Working with Universal Life Force Energy
Llyn Roberts, Robert Levy
Shamanism and Reiki are each powerful ways of healing; together,
their power multiplies. *Shamanic Reiki* introduces techniques to
help healers and Reiki practitioners tap ancient healing wisdom.
Paperback: 978-1-84694-037-8 ebook: 978-1-84694-650-9

Pagan Portals – The Awen Alone
Walking the Path of the Solitary Druid
Joanna van der Hoeven
An introductory guide for the solitary Druid, *The Awen Alone* will
accompany you as you explore, and seek out your own place
within the natural world.
Paperback: 978-1-78279-547-6 ebook: 978-1-78279-546-9

A Kitchen Witch's World of Magical Herbs & Plants
Rachel Patterson
A journey into the magical world of herbs and plants, filled with
magical uses, folklore, history and practical magic. By popular
writer, blogger and kitchen witch, Tansy Firedragon.
Paperback: 978-1-78279-621-3 ebook: 978-1-78279-620-6

Shapeshifting into Higher Consciousness
Heal and Transform Yourself and Our World with Ancient
Shamanic and Modern Methods
Llyn Roberts
Ancient and modern methods that you can use every day to
transform yourself and make a positive difference in the world.
Paperback: 978-1-84694-843-5 ebook: 978-1-84694-844-2

Readers of ebooks can buy or view any of these bestsellers by
clicking on the live link in the title. Most titles are published in
paperback and as an ebook. Paperbacks are available in traditional
bookshops. Both print and ebook formats are available online.

Find more titles and sign up to our readers' newsletter at
http://www.johnhuntpublishing.com/paganism
Follow us on Facebook at https://www.facebook.com/MoonBooks
and Twitter at https://twitter.com/MoonBooksJHP

You may also like…

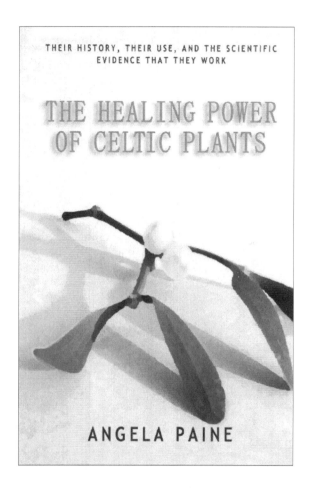

THEIR HISTORY, THEIR USE, AND THE SCIENTIFIC
EVIDENCE THAT THEY WORK

THE HEALING POWER
OF CELTIC PLANTS

ANGELA PAINE

The Healing Power of Celtic Plants
Their history, their use, the scientific evidence that they work

ISBN 978 1 90504 762 8

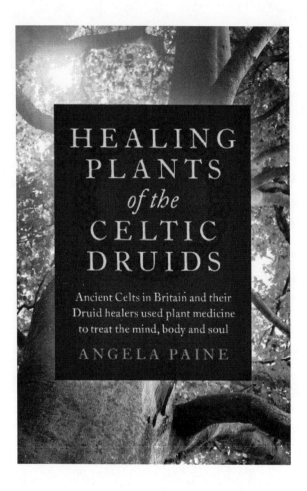

Healing Plants of the Celtic Druids

Ancient Celts in Britain and their Druid healers
used plant medicine to treat the mind, body and soul

ISBN 978 1 78535 554 7